Sustainable Community

A Framework for a Better Future

Wayne Fox

The Author does not assume any responsibility or liability whatsoever on behalf of the purchaser or reader of this material.

Any perceived slight of any individual or organization is purely unintentional. I sometimes use affiliate links with the content of the book. This means I will be paid a sales commission if you make a purchase. This, however, does not mean my opinion is for sale. Any affiliate links listed in the book are the services and products for which I've used myself and found beneficial. The reader or purchaser should do their research before making a purchase online.

Contents

What others are saying

Your reviews go here

Introduction

Sunday 12th March 2023. *'I can't feed my family, they've stolen my livelihood, I don't know what to do'*. Abayomi struggles to express her words choked up by her tears, not understanding how she can fix her situation. Until a few months ago, she'd scraped enough money together by selling souvenirs to tourists on the beach. Since then, the locals have been banned from accessing the beach.

Huge wire fences have been erected to stop them from visiting what was once their birthright. Her husband, Abdul, is a fisherman. He, too, can no longer earn a living; he no longer has access to the shoreline.

The hotel resorts in the local area have opened shops within their compounds; tourists have everything they need inside the resort. Few tourists explore the local area now; they're encouraged to buy everything they need from inside the resorts. Before this happened, Abayomi had survived on less than $45 a month to feed herself, her husband, and her five children. Her kids don't even have shoes to wear; they walk to school barefoot. Their school is small & cramped. During the rainy season, water cascades through the holes in the roof & onto the students. The building is in such a bad state of repair that any Western country would have abandoned it years ago, labelling it as a *'risk to life'*.

If any of Abayomi's family gets sick, there's no natural healthcare system to help them - just a makeshift hospital fifty miles away; Abayomi has no transport to reach it anyway. It's a similar story across many of the frontier and least developed countries. It's been this way for longer than I've been alive. Yet, many of these nations have some of the most valuable natural resources on the planet—gold, silver, diamonds, and oil. Suppose the wealth of a nation was a reflection of how valuable its natural resources were. In that case, these people should all be driving around in supercars. Yet, they struggle to buy the bare essentials for survival. This land belongs to the people, but a group of greedy parasites have stolen it.

Publishers always say you should have a target reader in mind when writing a book. The target reader, in this case, has to be me. Primarily, it's written for the freedom seeker in me, a rebel to the system, frustrated by the status quo in the world, hungry for drastic change for the sake of every human being on this planet.

It's for anyone who wants to create a better life for themselves and their family.

Secondly, this is for the many partners who can bring this framework to life. These can include hotel and spa operators wishing to grow and expand, along with the construction partners keen to lend their expertise and resources to witness the revolution happen.

Then there are the change makers, those who wish to impact people like Abayomi and her family by investing in a model that changes people's lives whilst earning a fantastic return on their investment.

My whole life has been in preparation for this time. I've been immersed for over 40 years in property development and construction. I'm the fourth generation of a family involved in construction and property development for the last 100 years, dating back to my great-grandfather, Fred Fletcher, a bricklayer from Nottingham, UK. I've been involved in many projects, from renovating old manor houses to building, fitting out and renovating hotels, offices, and housing estates.

During this time, I've learnt a lot about myself & what my strengths are. My ability to reignite a business, reimagine business models, and create new product offerings, combined with my ability to see the future & produce a vision that meets that future. These strengths have generated the most significant successes and frustrations in my life. I mention frustrations because when you tell someone a monster is coming over the hill, but they can't see or hear it, so they don't believe it's real. By the time they see it, it's too late. These last fifteen years have been filled with a lot of frustration as I repeatedly warned people only to witness their business die, & lose everything they'd worked so hard for their whole lives because they didn't believe the threat was real.

I first realized my strengths in my twenties, as we grew our family contracting business from a company working for a few local homeowners to a decade later having contracts & staff all over Scotland, working for many well-known customers, including Serco, Swallow Hotels & Best Western Hotels, along with many government local authorities. My partners have worked with firms like Disney, Four Seasons, & Marriott, as well as doing all kinds of exciting things, such as taking companies public.

In 2009, I got involved in a renewable energy start-up and, within two years, grew that to be the largest biomass energy company in the UK. A few years later, I got involved with a small media company, making about £200k annual revenue. Within four months, we'd secured a contract to export their services to China, worth over one million pounds. These are just two examples of the varied businesses I've reignited over the last three decades.

My focus now is on what I call *'the Freedom Revolution'*-—creating opportunities that lead us toward a healthier, opportunity-focused, and freedom-inspired world, which is some of what you'll read about in this book.

The reason for writing this book is to provide an understanding of where the world is heading and give a glimpse into an alternative way. I don't share this to fill your head with doom & gloom or conspiracy theories but rather so you can position yourself & your business so the coming tsunami of change & disruption doesn't affect you.

The bi-product of following this model, I'll share, is while you'll improve your own life and that of those around you, you'll also improve the lives of millions of people like Abayomi, who've been robbed of their birthright by the developed world, so a handful of greedy parasites can hoard their coin like a twisted evil golem creature, whilst those they've stolen from are left to rot, like dying rats.

I intend to provide you with a framework for improving different areas of your life, & I'll shine a spotlight on some areas you have yet to consider. Some suggestions might make you uncomfortable, leading you to dismiss them because they're so obvious you might question why you'd not discovered them before. By the end of the book, you'll have the foundations to build from, making changes in your own life whilst noticing the butterfly effect on everyone around you.

Our business intends to provide access to these alternative ways in a packaged format. We understand you live a busy life, and most might feel overwhelmed by this framework after reading through it. Others might want to be involved but must gain the direct skills or experience to know where to start.

Part of our immediate focus is to use our experience in property development and energy services, scaling businesses & raising investment to build a private village community, self-sufficiency solutions, hotel investment, hotel & spa developments, sustainable solutions for food, water, energy & waste, but ultimately use all these revenue generators to impact the lives of people like Abayomi & her family, which you'll read more about in part two.

The book is divided into two parts. Part one will examine the current issues in the system, what led to them, and where they will lead us if we don't wake up and change course quickly. In part two, I'll share our FREEDOM Framework™, providing seven areas to focus on, whether you want to improve your health or build your own community.

I start this journey with a simple question: *'What would it take to create a completely self-sustainable life—not just for me but for a community of people, each with their individual needs?'*

You can only see the view from Everest after first climbing the mountain. Good things come from uncomfortable situations. The climb starts right now.

Part One

The snake that feeds itself

This chapter will examine the world's current state, what led it to this point, and where it will end if we don't change course quickly. But I'm not about to start talking about climate change, as you might expect; that's how many of these *'sustainability books'* start.

This book is about moving away from those who push nefarious controlling agendas. As you read on, you'll understand why I say this. Humans are born free; they don't need to be dictated to by unelected bureaucrats. This chapter will discuss who these various agendas really benefit because, on the face of them, while they preach about saving the planet, most of them are about something much more nefarious. If you substituted the words *'climate change'* for *'ultimate control of the people,'* the same playbook would apply.

You must proceed cautiously if you have yet to see any of my trigger-inducing content before this point. In this section of the book, there's a strong chance something you read will trigger you & cause offence. This is a heads-up. I could have toned it down a bit to soften the blow, but the fact is, I'm not saying it to hurt anyone's feelings; it's not aimed at you, so remove yourself from the firing line and stop defending the system that shits on you. If you're offended by the truth I share, maybe ask yourself why you'd protect a system that continually makes you poorer, makes you sicker, makes you dumber, and ultimately makes you more reliant on it. If you're offended by it because you've spent a lifetime to qualify in a subject I'm about to shred, then I don't blame you for being upset. I would be, too, but I'm just the guy with the torch, trying to shine a light on the dark corridors of the system. It's the system you need to be angry with, not the guy with the torch.

Unfortunately, everywhere you look in the Western world, it's corrupt and toxic, mostly doing the opposite of what it's presented as. We live in an upside-down world where things presented as good are evil, while the real good things or people are presented as evil.

Suppose we're ever to find a sustainable solution to the problems in the world. In that case, we need to stop being offended by everything, stop taking everything so personally, forget all that brainwashing done to us, and start to live our lives in awareness of how the world really works. None of this will shock you if you're fully awake to everything I will share with you. Some of it might make you think even more deeply about how far this rabbit hole goes & why. So now I've prepared you mentally; it's time to get into it. Brace yourself.

Financial system

Did you know that in the Western world, 99.9% of businesses are small and medium-sized, yet less than 1% of investment goes into this part of the economy? The picture's even worse in frontier and least developed countries.

Most of the financial system is controlled, owned or dictated to by a small handful of investment funds & corporate interests. Blackrock, State Street & Vanguard have invested $22 trillion in the market. These aren't the only investment funds, but they own many of the assets in the market today. Every sector, whether it is public companies, pharmaceutical & technology companies, office space, social housing & farmland. This holding gives them a controlling influence on a large portion of the market and, with that, a substantial impact on how the world functions. The problem is more than just these three companies; numerous other controlling interests have existed much longer. Of course, we've always had our old friend *'Greed'*, which dominates everyone's mind at some point. I mention only these three significant investment funds as they're easy for you to research yourself if you want to, whereas other controlling parties are private.

As we witnessed in the 2008/09 financial crash, investment managers were incentivized to make deals regardless of whether they benefited the general public, the fund, or its investors.

The majority of the global economy is bankrupt. In the UK and US, the currency's value has lost over 90% in the last few years as governments continue printing fake money, devaluing their nation's wealth against other currencies. The global economy will eventually collapse, wiping out most people's savings, pensions, and wealth forever and probably taking every small business with it.

In 2020, the world experienced what some would call the corporate takeover of the global economy. While every small business in the Western nations was forced to shut down, the corporate monopolies were allowed to continue operating.

Why is it that the family-owned butcher shop on my village high street had to close, whilst the big supermarkets were okay to stay open? It makes sense once you realize everything was planned from the start. In my social media posts in 2018, I wrote that the plan was always to remove small businesses from the economy and have corporations dominate every industry.

Meanwhile, to avoid losing everything they owned, small business owners were forced to take on *'free money'* in the form of *'bounce back loans'*. Fast forward three years, and we have almost every business now laden with debt, each needing help to afford the repayments. In some cases, the interest rates on that debt are close to the same as a credit card. Many businesses have already ceased trading; every day, I see stories of more insolvencies, businesses that have traded for decades, household names, and small local businesses from my local area, all going insolvent.

Every business I speak to needs help paying their debt repayments. As the economy moves into recession, this downward spiral will speed up. As I write this in March 2024, I predict that by 2026, just two years from now, most small businesses will no longer exist in the Western economies.

Most people believe the money system was created as a form of value exchange. It was a way to exchange one hour of your time for a loaf of bread. That purpose is secondary. Money carries an energetic vibration; it represents *'flow'*, like water. We call it *currency*, like water has a current that will take a stick downriver. The problem is that the money system has been hijacked by a small group of nefarious characters in this play we call life.

The primary purpose of money now, rather than just being an exchange of value, is to control the mass population. It keeps people in the realm of seeking survival. The value the system currently rewards is anything that detracts people from their true essence or path, whether keeping them distracted or feeding them so much junk that they can't focus on what benefits them.

Exchange of value is great on a day-to-day basis for buying a loaf of bread or a pint of milk; these are basic survival needs, but what happens when we need more than survival?

Even the desire to take a holiday is limited by how much money we have. Do you want to learn a new subject? Gain a qualification? Improve your position in life? Buy a house? Take on a business project? It's all limited by your perception of having access to the money you need for those activities. But who controls your access to cash? It's the controllers of the system that keep you enslaved to it. It's the same people who created the current version of the monetary system.

The worst thing is that the central banks created all that debt from nothing. That money never existed in physical form. The current money supply is not backed by anything physical like precious metals, as it once was, because debt is created literally from nothing.

It's just digits on a screen that keep increasing when someone new borrows more money. If the funds were backed by physical gold bars, one bar of gold for, say, £1,000, it would be impossible for them to magically create debt from thin air, as there'd be no gold to back it up. If I want to lend you £10,000, I will go to my vault, remove the ten gold bars, and then pass them to you. If I didn't have those ten gold bars, I wouldn't be able to *'lend'* you that money.

The same principle applies to interest. Interest is a fictional number added to your debt and created from nothing. To pay me back that additional interest, you'd have to create new gold bars from somewhere, too, so I could then add them back to my vault, ready to lend again. Suppose there's a limited supply of gold in the system because it directly relates to how much currency is circulating. In that case, it's impossible to create more by magic. This was why the money supply was removed from the gold standard, to use it against the people.

Food system

Last year, after visiting the supermarket, I found a heavily bruised apple in my shopping bag. Rather than eat it myself, I threw it out into the garden for the birds to eat. The apple remained precisely as I'd thrown it out three months later. The birds hadn't touched it, and it was still as red as the day I'd thrown it out. Animals know what's healthy and what's not; they could see something wasn't right with this apple. What exactly are we putting in our bodies if it means it doesn't decompose naturally?

Enter the mainstream supermarkets; 95% of what they sell is toxic and poisonous to our bodies. I'm not talking about the typical junk food; that's obvious. I'm talking about those foods you believe are healthy for you. I'm talking about the fruit & vegetables sprayed with all sorts of chemicals. We'll understand why they tell us to *'eat our five a day'* later. Of course, this is all done to create a longer shelf life, which ultimately means the supermarkets can increase their profits.

Meanwhile, farmers who produce food to feed the population struggle to survive. Sometimes, they're paid just 1% of the actual retail price for the product. You might question how a farmer can feed 1,000 dairy cows when they're only paid a few pence for every litre of milk they produce. The fact is they cannot. Each year, farmers are losing money. Many have already sold their farms or diversified into other areas to use their land & resources better. A few have moved into selling directly to the local community, but this is a tiny fraction; it barely makes a dent in the overall community food supply, as most people continue to support these corporate parasites, rather than helping the food producers directly.

Many people buy canned food, such as tuna fish and baked beans. Canned food is intended to last as long as possible, so it is encased in airtight cans and filled with additives to extend its shelf life.

The problem with canned food, aside from all the additives, is that it leeches metals from the can, meaning when you eat that tin of baked beans, you're also ingesting those metals that your body can't digest.

Processed foods make up a large portion of the supermarket shelves. Even things like crab sticks, which you'd believe to be crab meat, have been processed with all sorts of rubbish added. Look at the ingredients of most of the food in this category, even things like chicken, and you'll find all kinds of fillers and other toxic trash added to it. These *'fillers'* are added to *'bulk-up'* the product, making it look bigger and weigh more. These are filler agents, gluten, soya, and Xanthan gum among others. Ingredients that most of us can't even pronounce. These are waste products that many people cannot digest; the sole purpose is to generate more profit for the supermarkets regardless of the health consequences to the people eating them.

I picked up a packet of *'turkey trimmings'* a few weeks ago whilst at the shop. This product was presented as pieces of turkey off-cuts. On looking at the ingredients, only 60% of the product was turkey. The rest comprised these fillers and other unnatural additives that shouldn't be in there. One of the fillers added was soya. Now, I could have unsuspectingly eaten this product expecting it to be 100% turkey, then suffered huge health repercussions as I'm allergic to soya. Soya is not a natural food source; it's a man-made food source created to feed cattle, fattening them up, ready for slaughter. So why are we now being fed it too... Perhaps they plan to slaughter us, too?

Another thing I've noticed in the past twelve months is the increasing amount of products containing Dextrose. Dextrose is a product which acts like sugar. I first learnt about Dextrose when a family member was diagnosed with type one diabetes. Dextrose is a fast-acting sugar substitute used by people with diabetes to rapidly increase their blood sugar levels when it's dangerously low.

It's sweet like sugar but acts much faster to raise blood sugar levels. So now you understand this: why are they putting it into our foods? Do you think there's any connection between the increasing number of people who have diabetes in the past decade?

Eating foods containing Dextrose will spike your blood sugar every time you eat. This impacts your pancreas, creating more insulin, which eventually will be under so much strain that it'll stop functioning correctly. At this point, you'll be reliant on pharmaceutical drugs to keep it under control. If later you have children, that weakness in your pancreas will be genetically passed onto your offspring, & they'll become type one sufferers.

Did you realize that artificial & non-caloric sweeteners like Aspartame, Sucralose, & Saccharine make you fat? Ironically, most people who consume these sweeteners, or *diet foods*, take them because they want the sweet taste without sugar calories. Aside from creating all sorts of health issues like migraines, sweeteners make your body crave sugar, so you consume more sugar from other places than you'd initially tried to save yourself from.

Water supply

Suppose you ever take a chemical sample of water from a household in a Western economy. In that case, you'll find large amounts of fluoride, chlorine, and other chemicals in the water. We're told these chemicals are used to kill parasites in the water. Yet, there are better, more efficient, and cheaper ways to kill any water-based parasites that don't involve poisoning the population of your country.

We should ask more profound questions of those we trust to provide our water supply. Is it worth considering if these chemicals are causing us health issues?

Health system

What are you thinking about if you're on a weight-loss diet and drinking protein shakes?!! Protein adds muscle. Muscle is heavier than fat. If you don't exercise and burn that extra protein, it'll become more fat. If you wish to lose weight, you don't eat bulk amounts of protein. If you look at anyone who goes through a diet plan, they might lose weight initially, but after they come off the plan, they always add more weight than they'd lost through the plan. Stop listening to the bell-ends that create these fad diet trends; they have one goal in mind - to keep you fat, so you'll continue buying their crap and listening to their bullshit.

If you're a fan of vitamins & supplements, I'm afraid I have even more bad news for you. Take a look at the ingredients in the supplements or vitamins. If it mentions an ingredient like *'magnesium stearate'*, this is used as what you might call a *'wrapper'*, which keeps it all together. The problem with this ingredient is that it prevents your body from absorbing the vitamins, so they swim around your body, never being absorbed. And then we wonder why people get all kinds of diseases like cancer.

But this leads us to the reason, besides profit, why things are the way they are: the pharmaceutical industry or, more broadly, the medical system.

Millions of people are employed in the *'cancer industry'*- research, treatment or aftercare services. Imagine how much money companies and their shareholders make in this fight. Now, imagine one of these lab technicians accidentally stumbled across an overnight cure for cancer. How many people and businesses would be unemployed within months of discovering this cure? You take a tablet and never get cancer again. If you were lucky to find the cure, you might be motivated to cover it up. Wouldn't you? If not you, you're seniors in the organization, those responsible for generating massive shareholder returns. You've got a family to feed and a new house to pay for; what about that lifestyle you've become accustomed to? Besides, you've spent your whole life working on this; what job would you do next? Do you even have the skills to get a new job? Would you like to showcase this discovery and become unemployed next month? It may be better just to bury it.

You might say certain parts of the industry are more motivated to actually 'grow' cancer cases, as this *'guarantees'* that you can maintain that lifestyle; you might even get a pay rise. But how might you increase cases?

One route is to feed people processed food and tell them to *'eat your five a day'*, consuming fruit and vegetables filled with all sorts of toxic chemicals. Or you could give them tablets for their IBS or Acid reflux, which, over time, creates further complications. Does the idea still seem unbelievable?

You might say it all sounds a bit *'conspiracy theory'* until you see evidence of it happening. A few years ago, Johnson & Johnson was found guilty of putting asbestos & arsenic into babies talcum powder. What a novel idea, a pharmaceutical company putting a harmful ingredient into a product, & worse still, by doing it to customers at the earliest & weakest stage in their immune system development; those babies grow up suffering all kinds of health issues. Allergies, right through to cancer, therefore guaranteeing future demand for drugs from the same industry that created the problem. It doesn't matter to these organizations if they get fined billions of dollars for doing it, because those customers they've *'infected'* with their poison are worth many trillions over their lifetime as a customer to the industry. A few billion dollars in fines is pocket change in the big scheme. It's like giving them a slapped wrist and calling them naughty boys and girls.

The traditional medical system (allopathic) is not trained to find the root cause of your health symptoms. It's trained to diagnose the symptom, then prescribe a medication which suppresses that symptom, making you believe you're cured, whilst, in reality, the real cause of the problem still exists, slowly manifesting something much bigger. Whilst it takes away one symptom, a few months later, fresh symptoms appear, maybe in the form of aches and pains or sniffles somewhere else in the body. When people have a cough, cold, or even the flu, this is just your body's natural method of getting rid of those toxins you've ingested. By taking all these medications, people suppress those sniffles and prevent their bodies from *'throwing out the trash'*.

What would happen if you never threw out the trash in your house, instead just letting it build up? Eventually, it would attract rodents, and you'd have many new problems. Why would it be any different with your own body?

This symptom suppression leads to the situation most people over 40 find themselves in. They take so many medications that you can probably hear them rattling as they walk up the street. Most of these medications become long-term prescriptions, with the doctor never reassessing the patient & removing them from the medication. They continue prescribing the drug for the rest of the patient's life. There's a good reason for this happening, as we'll get into next.

In 2018, I attended a business seminar in London, where I met a man named Simon. I talked to Simon, who told me he owned a string of NHS doctors and dental surgery businesses. He told me he was looking for more of these businesses to buy; I believe he had seven practices at the time. I'm not talking about owning the physical buildings; I'm talking about the actual operating business.

Until then, I believed all NHS surgeries were owned and run by the government. That is not the case; they're owned and run privately, generally by the doctors who work in them, and so we have a dilemma when we know how these *'businesses'* get paid.

 The doctors get paid money from the pharmaceutical companies every time they prescribe a medication from that company. They're unofficial salespeople. There's an apparent conflict of interest. This doesn't bode well for someone we trust to work in our best interests. Nor does it motivate the individual to find the root cause of our problems, as that would remove any future *'revenue'* from the customer for these drug pushers.

But we haven't finished yet. Bear with me. If you're a visiting alien to this planet, reading this, you'll probably think, *'Wow, what a crazy place. Why would people unquestioningly trust these parasites to take care of their health for them?'*

If we look into the health & hygiene aisle at the supermarket, we see products that are full of chemicals and are bad for our bodies. Most people don't realize this, but look at any of the ingredients in things like toothpaste, soap, shampoo, and makeup. Suntan lotion, for example, actually contains metallic particles that attract heat from the sun.

If wearing factor 50 is what saves us from skin cancer, then why isn't everyone in the hot, sun-drenched developing world already dead? They don't wear Factor 50. Buying this stuff would cost more than they earn in wages. But where is the skin cancer epidemic at its worst? It's Western countries that coat themselves in this toxic poison. The skin is the body's largest organ; every time we use these poisons & potions, they're absorbed by our skin, & into our bloodstream.

Let's briefly consider anything you put on your skin from these mainstream corporations, including moisturizers, makeup and even those *'natural'* products. Again, please look at the ingredients, but instead of searching and being deceived by words you can't pronounce, look at what those ingredients do to your body. What if I told you those *'age reduction'* creams make your skin age faster? How can that be so? One reason is that the products contain petroleum or paraffin-based ingredients.

Would it seem normal for you to rub your whole body with diesel? Of course, it wouldn't, but you do this every time you rub these *'skin care'* products all over your body. It's the same core product. These ingredients dry out your skin, reinforcing your need to buy the product you believe will fix the problem, getting you stuck in this cycle of buying more of the very thing that's causing you the trouble.

A few years ago, there was a massive movement against makeup products being tested on animals. Still, nobody seemed to question: If the product was *'natural'* and good for your skin, why did they need to test it on animals in the first place? Indeed, we missed a big red flag there. We should have asked what chemicals they were putting into these products when we witnessed the harm to these poor animals.

Technology

The intention has always been to create reliance on *'personal devices and technology'*. The system's controllers aim to connect everyone's body and brain to a vast computer network. This will be sold to you as a solution to make us smarter - imagine having all the world's information as an extension of your brain. At first, it sounds interesting, but we still need to consider its downside.

Imagine how easy it is for someone to hack into your computer at home. Now imagine how easy it is for someone to hack into that giant *'connected brain'*. A hacker could control an entire population at the click of a button, creating an army if they chose to. If we were meant to have computers for brains, we'd have them in-built when we pop out of the womb. These people are pushing this technology because a connected brain can be easily controlled or switched off. They can terminate our program if they choose to.

The transition from the early-stage mobile phone into this fully-fledged connected brain is slow. It's purposely slow, so we don't notice the transition & start questioning the intention.

The first step was creating a handheld computer device - the modern-day smartphone. We become reliant on this for everything in our day-to-day life; we have our work information on it, our banking & finances on it, and our life has become dependent

46

on it, so much so that if it's misplaced, we have a panic attack.

The next stage in this transition is *'wearable technology'*. This 'smart technology' moves from our hands to being fixed to our bodies. Smart technology includes earbuds, smart watches, and other *'health'* monitoring devices. It also consists of the glasses that have recently been released. Note how all these devices are connected to the internet's central network. We're now just one step away from connecting our brains to the network.

If you look at the so-called *'heroes'* like Elon Musk, he's connected a human brain to a computer with his business, Neuro-link. He also has a vast global satellite network called Star-Link, which, when the brain is connected, will ensure everyone remains connected to the internet, regardless of where they are. It is complete control of the human race.

Now, I need to express massive concern. This wearable technology is more than just the smart devices mentioned above. These are for the mainstream, but other *'devices'* are already out there, being relied on in different sectors of the economy. The medical devices industry creates wearable technology, whether diabetes monitors, insulin pumps, or prosthetic limbs. I know it is challenging if you already use these, but be careful about what you become reliant on. With this technology, we must return to basics rather than moving closer to a connected brain solution.

Take the insulin pumps, for example; these are already connected to the internet via a smartphone. If the controller wanted to, they could tap into that device while you sleep and alter how much insulin it gives you. It sounds far-fetched when I say this right now, but the next evolution of these devices will enable them to do that easier than ever. It's a straightforward way for the system controllers to keep you reliant on them.

When you're reliant, you're also compliant. At that point, there's no turning back.

Charity

Charities are run for the benefit of those who create or run them. I can't lump every charity into this category as I have yet to research all of them. Still, looking at the more significant, well-known charities, I'll make some blanket statements based on what appears to be everyday actions across many of them.

There's a lot I can say about the charity sector. Still, until the news is shared publicly, it'll just attract libel cases from large donors and benefactors as they scramble to avoid the information becoming public knowledge. So, until that time, I can only share what's already in the public realm, albeit hidden in some regards.

Did you know a scam has been running in charities for at least a decade? I first heard about it in 2013, and I'm sure it wasn't anything new back then. An individual or a business donates money to the charity. The charity will then pay them back 90% of that donation as an income or by giving a fake contract to the donor company. Whilst the charity keeps 10% of the donation (plus 25% gift aid claimed from the government), the 90% paid back to the donor is classed in the charity's financial accounts as a *'cost of raising funds'*. By donating, the donor can claim it as a tax-deductible expense, which means they'll pay much less tax on their income & profits. But then they also earn extra income the following year, as the donation gets returned to them..... and we haven't even started on the big boys yet.

A well-known global charity, it goes by the name of *'Oxfam',* you might have heard of it. Over the past decade, it faced numerous charges against the senior management for not investigating reports that its staff were raping children in developing countries. In another case, senior management had visited a developing country & for several weeks, had trafficked young girls, held them captive during their trip to the country, and had sex with them. This charity presents itself as being against child trafficking and sex slavery.

There are a few smaller charities with pure intentions, run by good, honest people who work tirelessly and voluntarily without pay.

Unfortunately, the actions of the corrupt and the evil intent of the well-known charity brands will tarnish the image of *'charity'* overall, so these smaller, good-intentioned charities will suffer for it, too.

Housing system

The final thing I wish to shed some light on is how we live in this world, specifically these places we call our homes. Have you ever noticed that when you travel to a particular place, you feel a certain way about it? I'm susceptible to this, so I can quickly feel what a place is like.

The reason we have high crime & violence in dense areas of a city is because any negative emotions or energy are magnified. Suppose you've ever walked into a room after an argument, & felt an atmosphere in the room, or walked into a place where all the people in the room have been crying. In that case, you pick up a feeling of sadness from the room. If you stayed in that place, you'd start to feel those emotions as if they were your own.

If one person is angry in a block of apartments, the rest of the flats around them also start to feel angry, despite not knowing why they feel this way.

The same applies to dense areas of a city. The other reason these areas generate high crime & violence is similar to when you cage a lion in a small space; it becomes frustrated and angry. Like the lion, you are not meant to be enclosed in this small space we call home.

We're meant to live in open plains in nature, not in tightly compacted concrete jungles with no breathing space. Humans are not designed to live in this small concrete box, so this frustration builds & impacts how you think and act. Suppose your windows look toward the open landscape, toward nature. In that case, your mindset will be very different than if it views the dirty concrete jungle.

Our environment dictates how we think and act. Areas of dense social housing have been purposely designed with this in mind. The system's 'controllers' don't want you to become an enlightened being because then you'd realize that you don't need them to survive in this world.

Instead, they keep you in the fight-or-flight survival mode.

Interestingly, this mass development of so-called *'Tiny Homes'* has occurred over the last two years. Do they not understand we're not meant to be confined in small spaces like these? Or are they just profiting off society regardless of the health consequences for those who buy them?

A *'Tiny Home'* is, in some cases, smaller than the size of a 20ft shipping container. I wonder if the creators choose to live in a shipping container themselves or whether they prefer a lovely manor house in the country. What has our world become when we care more about profit than providing something of value to the customer?

Go to any corporate property developer and pay £500,000 to live in a tiny box with a matchbox garden, & overlooked by five other tiny boxes around it, designed to squeeze as many small boxes into the space as possible to increase profit. Does that seem like something you'd get into a lifetime of debt for? This is what most people in Western society aspire toward.

When we consider the construction of our homes, & workspaces, the materials used in the construction & furnishing of these buildings are toxic & poisonous to our health. Many of the modern world's construction methods create mould & dampness and other conditions such as SAD (seasonal affective disorder) syndrome. The paint on the walls contains VOCs (Volatile Organic Compounds), which poison us. Formaldehyde is in almost every building material, as well as being in our furnishings & floor coverings. Our homes & workspaces are poisoning us every single day.

Please consider the effects of Wi-Fi networks on our bodies, too; Wi-Fi emits electromagnetic frequencies into our homes, disrupting the function of our internal organs. That's not the worst of it, though.

Every time you live in a building that's been dug into the rock, such as digging a basement level into the ground or encasing the building in stone, the rock emits radon into the building and causes cancer. When living near electricity pylons, the radon becomes very sticky, speeding up the onset of cancerous tumours in our bodies. This information has been known in the mainstream for over thirty years, but the world has continued to build using this method. These buildings should be demolished.

The Climate change agenda

In the past four years, I've been censored and shadow-banned on social media, so much so that you've probably not read any of my posts or watched any of my videos. For those who have, you might have believed me to be some *'climate change denier'*. This isn't true. I've yet to study the data, but I know it's easy for someone to manipulate it to provide the exact answer you want people to see.

There's also confirmation bias, where our brain will always find evidence to back up our beliefs on a particular subject, so if we've been brainwashed by the media, movies and other PR campaigns to have certain beliefs about a topic, our brain will search out evidence to confirm that belief.

What I don't like about the climate change narrative is how a bunch of bureaucrats tell me I have to live a certain way, I must pay lots of extra hidden taxes and carbon levies, and these thieving parasites fly to Switzerland to a *'climate change summit'*, each flying in their private jets and helicopters, paid for by the taxpayer. In Davos, Switzerland, each year for a few weeks, there are over 300 jets parked up on an airfield, carrying bureaucrats that lie to us & instruct us *'normal people'* that we must cut back our carbon footprint. The irony is unreal.

Meanwhile, these bureaucrats receive untold riches from those corporate fat cats, who benefit when people comply with the latest 'carbon reduction measures'. I'm talking about the type of company that can increase its prices, using *'carbon taxes'* as its excuse. Those corporate manufacturers create energy technologies, such as solar panels, battery packs, and electric vehicles, while parading it under this PR campaign called *'sustainability'*.

They don't care about sustainability; it's about filling their pockets with your money. It's one big tax scam.

Is the human race in trouble if it doesn't change its ways? Yes. Look at the vast craters being created on the earth to dig up a few precious metals, all to feed the greed of a small group of people. Who is it that benefits from mining these rare & precious metals?

Did you realize there are probably more diamonds in the world than chocolate bars? Only you don't see them because those who own the diamond mines, such as the Oppenheimer family, hold back all diamonds in vaults to prevent them from flooding the market. They're about as rare as a grain of sand.

 But whilst people continue to pay exorbitant amounts of money for this stuff, these ruling families will continue to dig up the earth, leaving these vast craters in their wake. I recommend you watch a movie called *'Blood Diamond'*. It might change your mind about the diamond industry. The colour of the stone might change, but the same remains true. It's all for the benefit of a few greedy parasites. Are you starting to notice a theme yet?

So much *'greenwashing'*, *'carbon washing'*, or *'sustainability washing'* is being bandied about. Still, most of it is just an excuse to either sell more to you, increase prices, or pretend some are better than others, with all their virtue signalling. Sell you more stuff you never needed to *'save the planet'*. It's the same playbook with a different front cover.

Ask most people who push these *'sustainability'* narratives what sustainability means, & they won't know the true answer. They'll probably say it's about reducing carbon emissions or some other bullshit like that. A sustainable process, or system, creates more than it consumes without detracting from other systems.

Government

Until the last few years, most people believed that only the developing countries in Africa had corrupt governments. In recent years, we've also seen how corrupt our Western governments are. They award *'special favours'* to their friends and create *'furlough'* schemes so their families can claim millions in *'free money'*.

They awarded *'fast track'* contracts worth hundreds of millions to their peers in the House of Lords. We had the government boffins going on live TV threatening forced vaccinations, which, of course, benefited their parasite mates in the pharmaceutical industry. I hope these people enjoy their comfortable prison cell, when the people realize how much they were screwed over. Was the money worth it?

Anyone who still believes they need someone else to make decisions on their behalf should be careful about whom they give that responsibility. Someone else might pay them handsomely to make decisions that don't suit your best interests.

Your local politician, Jimmy, the ex-grocer from your high street, will never have a hope in hell's chance of being inside that inner circle that controls the political party's actions. It's all designed this way. You cannot fix the problem by voting for a different colour necktie. They're just two sides of the same coin. For those who believe they can stand for some nondescript local *freedom party'*, ask yourself if you can make a difference and stand a hope in hell of forming a government.

Firstly, in the UK, you need to have 600 local MPs running in their local constituencies, spending millions on putting out your political story to the public. Otherwise, your chance of forming a government is next to zero. In this case, do you wish to change the system, or is it an exercise to raise your own profile? When you vote for Jimmy, you're voting to keep the corrupt parasites in play.

In Latin, *'Government'* means *'Control the mind'*. We live in a world where the government controls our minds, presenting us with all kinds of perceptions about how things are so it can control us. A vote for any government is a vote FOR government. Any form of traditional government is not in the people's best interest.

Education

A system where we send our kids to prison camps for twenty years so they can learn how to be compliant slaves & robots. Imagine a world where we sit in a classroom memorizing irrelevant nonsense that we'll never think about or need again.

The current education system is so removed from the real world that it's unfathomable how we ever accepted it being okay to teach this nonsense to us.

After completing the first part of the prison sentence, which we call high school, we volunteer for a second sentence, where we build up huge debts whilst memorizing more irrelevant rubbish that we'll never use in the real world. Stupid things like correctly referencing an essay using the *'approved Harvard referencing format'*. Have you ever heard such a lot of bullshit like this before?

If you're a university graduate, you probably never questioned it. Well, now, I'm here to question it for you and bring it to the front of your consciousness so you, too, can ask why.

Now, I mention this example because whilst I didn't attend university, in 2007, I started a distance learning university course. After spending two months studying a subject every hour of my spare time, evenings and weekends. I submitted my first two assessments for grading. The lecturer returned them immediately, and both were graded as a *'fail'*. He'd failed them because I needed to correctly reference the essays in the Harvard-approved format. See, the system didn't care what I'd written in those essays; the lecturer told me the content was correct, but he'd failed the essays because the system cares more about me complying with it than being correct & factual.

After being free of the school system for over ten years by this point, I wasn't about to get back into being compliant, so I told them to stick the course up their arse.

Take my nephew as another example; just like myself & many other people, he is not suited to the academic system a system where we get rewarded for how good we are at memorizing and regurgitating irrelevant nonsense, & so his time at high school has been a struggle as far as getting *'good'* grades. In one of his math lessons, he complained that he couldn't understand how to do it. To punish his lack of understanding, they put him in detention. Of course, this didn't solve the problem; he still didn't understand how to do it.

His example work in his math class was called an inverted fraction. If you're like me & you've never seen one before, you'll probably ask what the hell these things are used for in the real world. I left school 30 years ago, and I never saw an inverted fraction in my time at school; I've never seen one since leaving school, nor have I come across any opportunity in the real world where I'd get the chance to use one. All I can imagine is this stuff has been created by a *'bell-end boffin'* to make them feel clever. It's a pity they didn't dedicate their life to creating something worthwhile.

There's a reason that 99% of the most successful people left school without qualifications. It's a direct correlation. It's because they couldn't grasp the pointless system of compliance, learning stuff that had no connection to the real world. They didn't become reliant on irrelevant rubbish so that they could function in real life. They maintained their ability to think for themselves.

The Reason

On a spiritual level, the universe has orchestrated certain events to show us how these systems don't serve us and to free humanity from its caveman existence and mindset.

The system has been this way for centuries to keep people operating at this survival level, keeping people in the reactive fight or flight mode. This keeps them trapped in a nefarious debt cycle, shackled to a job they hate, disconnected from their purpose, and living in a state of depression, as their soul craves something more from their existence, all to maintain their ego's need to hold onto these shiny objects. To the uninitiated, this sounds like the crazy ramblings of a madman. Still, if you're reading this book, your soul resonates with it at some level.

From birth, we're fed a constant stream of brainwashing, telling us we *need* this item or that for us to feel sexy, successful, beautiful, wanted, part of the tribe, complete, etc. We need that new BMW 3 series; we need that white picket-fenced suburban house with its tiny rooms & zero character. The same applies to cars, homes, holidays, mobile phones, or that designer-label baby's pram. If we don't have these *things*, our social circle might think less of us.

We're told we must live our lives walking down a particular path. We must go to school & learn how to comply with authority figures, then go to university and memorize information we'll never

need for a job that won't exist in ten years,
eventually being replaced by robots & automation.

We should get married and have two kids, buy the latest gadgets, buy a house in suburbia, go to watch the football on a Saturday, drink and be merry every weekend - drowning our sorrows for a life we hate but have no way out of, shackled by the debt we've taken on, for the life we thought we wanted. We should work a 9 to 5 for the rest of our miserable lives, then retire, living in poverty, waiting to die. We're told to save for a rainy day, putting off *'life'* until retirement because travelling the world is for old-aged pensioners. The only problem with that premise is that when we retire, our joints are so brittle that it's a struggle to climb out of bed, never mind climb a mountain. Anyone choosing a life that doesn't precisely match every part of this playbook is ridiculed by society, viewed as a failure, or a *'weirdo'* for not going with the norm.

This path is only presented as *'normal'* because it saddles you with the shackles of debt. If you have debt, you must repay the borrowed money to maintain that shiny lifestyle. More importantly, if you're indebted to someone, you're easy to control, whether you're an individual, a business, or an entire country.

Conclusion

In a utopian society, everyone could access capital to take on a project and start or grow a business. Nobody would live on the streets, and we would all have the resources we need: food, water, shelter, somewhere to live, access to capital, energy, and, most importantly, a purpose.

The perception of having access to money limits and controls us as a population. Those who control the money supply create it from thin air. It's just numbers on a screen. To learn more about that, look into the fraud they call *'fractional reserve banking'*. If I created my own notes and coins, telling people it was money, I'd get thrown in prison, yet this bunch of mobsters do, and the people just let them.

For the human race to escape survival mode, we must collectively shift from perception to reality because that's how they control us. You perceive their systems to be serving your highest and best interests, but the truth is that they're just in place to control you.

What will you say to your grandkids when they ask what role you played during *'The Great Cull'* of the 21st century? For most, the answer will probably be, *'Oh well, kids, the reason your life is so rubbish, the reason you're a slave to the system, is because we stood by and let it happen. A few crazy people were shouting about how corrupt the government was, but we just mocked and ridiculed them. We wish we'd paid more attention and helped them change things; oh well, bad luck, kids; you can live in a world we created through our inaction against those who enslave you now.*

Watch the *Lord of the Rings* movie trilogy. You'll probably remember the little *'Golem'* character if you've seen it. He was the one who followed the hobbits, trying to steal the ring from them. Whilst you believed it was all just fiction, the *Lord of the Rings* story reflects the human journey through life. We're heading for the ultimate battle between good and evil, just like the hobbits had to face at the end of their quest. Golem represents the greedy parasites that will do anything to gather more coins. There's no purpose to them doing it other than collecting as many coins as possible.

You might think that I prefer socialism and I'm anti-capitalist. This is not the case. Socialism will never be good for humanity. Handing more money and power to those who created the problem is not the way out of this mess. There needs to be a rapid shake-up around how we reward value creation.

In this part of the book, we've highlighted some of the significant issues with the parasitical systems running the world. If you feel drawn to go down any of those rabbit holes to learn more about the problem, I'd encourage you to do that. I spent many years immersed in looking at the problem, but now I'm focused on creating the solution instead. I'm more interested in creating a better way for the human race to thrive outside of these parasitical systems so that my kids and those that follow them can have a better world than the one we live in today. A place where citizens don't have to worry about having somewhere to live, worrying whether they can afford to switch their heating on, constantly getting sick because of the food they consume, or doing a job they hate, shackled to a mountain of debt. In part two, I'll share our vision for a better future, & a plan to help everyone get there.

I think Michael Jackson sang, 'The children are our future, let them shine, and let them lead the way'. The children are the human race. But if we aren't willing to change anything, I feel sorry for the children that come after you. I can only pray these future generations have a bit more backbone & fight about them than the generations alive today.

All I see is a nation of pathetic, weak & feeble people, happy to roll over in favour of their *'comfortable life'*. Isn't it time you grew a set of balls and stood up against the very people that try to screw you over? If not, I suggest you bend over and lube up because you're in for a rough ride.

For those few who are ready to change things, I will share my initial thoughts on a framework for change. I call this the Freedom Framework, a framework for a better future.

Part Two

Framework for a better future

The *'circular economy'* concept has recently entered the mainstream narrative. The problem with this proposed solution is that it seems to focus heavily on reusing other people's junk—the idea is to avoid landfill by giving it to someone else.

That's a great idea if someone wants or needs it. There's nothing wrong with that idea, but it only looks at a small piece of a broken system. It's looking at mass consumerism as the blame for all the world's problems.

Passing our unwanted items to someone else pushes the problem down the road. If I give away my old clothes, I need to buy more clothing from somewhere else, & as these items don't last forever, at some point, I need to buy them new. At some time in the future, those items I gave away will become worn out. Eventually, they'll hit the landfill pile, so it's not a circular economy.

In a sustainable circular economy, those old trousers would either last forever or be repurposed into something completely different, which would either last forever or later be repurposed again. Their usefulness would never die.

In this section, I want to share a vision for a real circular economy, a sustainable way to live, run our business, and thrive in our community. I call this the framework for a better future. The FREEDOM Framework™ is a seven-step methodology.

Formula: Formula is focused on the overall business model for change, & for achieving the objective of our plan.

Root: Root is focused on the foundations of our society, & what's needed to make it work.

Exchange: Exchange focuses on what we perceive as our *'economy'* and alternative ways to exchange value.

Energize: Energize is about attracting the financial resources needed to make your master plan come to life.

Design: Design is focused on the parts required within a community structure to make it a success.

Optimized: Optimized is about the infrastructure & pieces that go into our community, from the energy services to the physical buildings

Mortal: Mortal is about the Human, & building our body into a picture of health

Formula

This chapter will examine an alternative model for life—a business model that can meet all our needs while creating opportunities for millions worldwide and lifting them out of poverty.

About twelve months ago, I watched a video about someone who'd built a school in Uganda, & how much it'd impacted the local people. Along with building a school, they also built an orphanage & created a freshwater supply.

Some kids didn't have shoes; they'd walk through the jungle barefoot. So they gave everyone new shoes too. By the end of that ten-minute video, I was uncontrollably crying, but I had no idea why. Every time I saw how grateful the people were for being helped, I'd get another burst of emotion. I know this is what I'm meant to work on. I knew this was the answer to that question I'd been searching for the last twenty years, the reason I was put on this planet. But let me rewind a bit to give you some context of how we got here.

In 2007, I became interested in helping those less fortunate. I didn't know what, who or where at the time, but in this instance, it was helping kids in Ghana. When I came across their story, something ignited a feeling I cannot explain: a sense of intense emotion. It was a time in my life when I felt lost. There must be a more significant reason for me being on this planet, other than just the hamster wheel existence. While I liked my role in our business, the thought that I'd still be doing the same thing until I die felt pointless.

Since 2002, I'd believed there must be a higher purpose or reason for us being, but I didn't know what that purpose was, so I'd been searching for it ever since.

I am trying to remember how it came to be. Still, I came into contact with a charity that renovated schools in Ghana. According to the charity, these kids were studying in buildings that were falling apart. There were holes in the floor, holes in the walls, holes in the roof. As soon as I saw it, I had this emotional connection inside my heart, knowing I was meant to be involved. I knew straight away, with my experience in the construction industry, building & renovating buildings, I could make a significant impact on these people very quickly.

The charity was accepting volunteers to make the repairs. Most of the volunteers were gap-year students. Still, with my combined construction and business experience, I immediately thought I could transform how this charity operated to make a more significant impact. Each volunteer paid £8,000 per week, which covered the cost of buying building materials, food, water, and accommodation with a local family in Ghana.

The cost was steep. I've been in the construction industry my whole life, and I know building materials don't cost that much, especially in developing countries. My conversations with the guy running the charity led me to conclude, the whole thing was a scam designed to catch the wealthy gap-year crowd. With some regret, I put the idea on the back burner, as I couldn't find any other organizations with the same objectives.

Fast forward fifteen years to 2022, I had an idea to convert a 1000-acre estate on the South coast of England into a five-star hotel resort & private village. It was a £100m project;

I had all the pieces in place to make it happen: the money, the operator, and the land; the only pieces I didn't have were the people to deliver the project. - the architect, the construction company, etc. Every firm I spoke to said they weren't interested, *we don't work with new customers'*, or *'come back in twelve months, we're too busy'*. At the time, this frustrated me a lot. I've experienced this attitude from contractors in the UK for three decades, but this was the worst ever. The attitude towards opportunity in the UK is a topic for discussion in another book, but this meant the proposed project couldn't proceed. I now believe this was the universe's way of pushing me toward the correct path—the path I now find myself on.

We all want to thrive in life, yet few people do. Most of the world's economy is controlled by the corporate sector. You buy food from supermarkets, travel in public transport, or buy vehicles and fuel from large corporations. Every time we buy something, we send our money out of the local economy; from then on, it never returns.

Only when that money continues circulating in that local economy can we thrive.

You might argue that these corporate entities, based thousands of miles away, employ local people. That's great, but these employees are generally minimum-wage earners. If you dig deeper, these workers' actual income, also considering taxes and other deductions, is less than 5% of the money you've spent with that business. This is a poor return for society.

Those workers then go and buy or rent a house, and somewhere in that property chain, there's a strong chance there'll be a corporate house builder that created it. They'll buy a car from a global car manufacturer. They buy energy from an international energy company. They'll take on debt, mortgages, car loans, and credit cards, paying exorbitant amounts of interest to worldwide corporations. The system is designed to take money out of the local economy because that creates a need for you to borrow even more.

Don't think I'm innocent in this whole game for a second. I've been on all sides of this debate: the consumer, the borrower, and the company. For much of my career, I focused on operating contrary to the model I'll discuss later. In our first business, a contracting business based in Scotland, UK, we would take on contracts that were hundreds of miles away from our office where we were based. Most of the time, staff travelled from another area to service those contracts. After that, I built a renewable energy business, which became the largest biomass company in the UK, again delivering contracts nationally but based in the north of Scotland, hundreds of miles from the customer. The universe took me down this path to make me aware of how damaging the process was for those local economies.

I could never talk about it if I'd not lived both sides of it myself.

Some people wouldn't like me saying this, but charity doesn't work. It's not sustainable. If I give a million pounds to charity, when it's gone, it's gone. That money will impact someone's life, but when the money's gone, it's gone forever. To make the same impact again, we need to find someone else to take another million pounds and do the same again. Eventually, the money is completely spent. It's a zero-sum game; it never comes back.

Charity also creates a reliance economy, or reliance mindset, where one person becomes reliant on another for their needs. But what happens when that provider can no longer provide?

One of my skills is imagining different business models for operating a business, so this problem got me thinking. This was just a business model problem. I needed to create a model that wasn't a zero-sum game. I needed to imagine a model that generated recurring income without relying on one person to donate the money.

Around the time of reaching my peak frustration in 2022, I started to see more and more evidence & news from African countries, despite, at the time, my complete dismissal of Africa as somewhere I should go for a business project. I spoke to an Ethiopian expat living in the UK, who suggested I invest in projects in Ethiopia. I never considered Ethiopia as a potential business opportunity, mainly because of the Western media brainwashing. I then started getting many random people from Africa to message me on social media, asking if I could sponsor their education so they could finish school.

I'd see videos on my YouTube newsfeed of investment incentives for various African countries despite never searching for them. It was at this point that I eventually started to investigate deeper.

Around the same time, I was also researching alternative ways of living. Alternative communities & off-grid living, so I started to wonder if I could build an off-grid alternative community in Africa.

I'd researched the communities already being constructed. Still, they always felt like by joining one of these communities, I'd be sacrificing basic comforts. I pictured hanging my laundry to dry on tree branches and living like *'tree people'*. Rather than the idea of going back to nature, these communities took the idea even further; it felt more like going back to being a caveman. That's different from my idea of living in an *'alternative community'*. Why does living outside of the mainstream systems have to mean you sacrifice comfort?

While researching alternative communities, I couldn't imagine myself living there. The idea of everyone sitting around a big dining table, cooking each other's meals, living in each other's pockets didn't gel with my thinking. I don't believe the people who first imagined this concept have lived in close proximity to people for an extended period themselves. For this reason, I think many of these communities will not succeed in the long term.

People are too dissimilar. Even people with the same interests today will grow apart in the future, so being forced to live in close proximity, cooking each other's food & living out of each other's pockets, whilst it might seem an exciting idea in the short term, it won't survive the future split.
 I've heard of people joining such communities to spend the rest of their lives there, only to leave less than two years later.

I'm attracted to living on a private island away from people. I mean no disrespect to anyone, but being huddled around the dining table makes my skin crawl. I prefer to be isolated, with just a small group around me. I need my personal space. So, I started to look into more traditional gated communities, & I found a company that builds standalone high-end communities for high-profile celebrities. These communities have dedicated village facilities and armed security guards at every gate. Properties in these communities typically sell for between £10m - £25m.

Still, suppose you're a Hollywood movie star or an ex-president and want privacy. In that case, this type of community is perfect.

Whilst a community like this is excellent, it also has a downside. It carries steep running costs, which comes back to what we said earlier about reducing that long-term financial commitment. The cost to maintain these 500-acre private villages, along with all the facilities and staff, is divided across 400 homes in the village, meaning each homeowner pays more than £50,000 annually in fees.

While I'd discovered the type of community that would fit my personal needs, the overall model didn't work how I'd planned. I completely understand why the concept I share here would not work in their communities.

A Profit-For-Purpose vehicle

There's a concept that'll seem foreign to most.

'All of your income should be invested at the source to provide returns that pay for your living expenses.'

Suppose you calculate your living expenses to be £100,000 a year. We'll assume an average return on our investments to be 10%. Without considering taxes, if our living expenses are £100,000 per year, at a 10% average return, we'd invest £1,000,000 into assets that generate that 10% return. Subsequently, this would pay for our living expenses. More importantly, we'd still have the original £1,000,000 capital, sitting across various investments, and those returns would keep flowing to us every year from that point forward. Now we understand this concept, let's go deeper.

The problem we're trying to solve here is to help local people. The original reason for doing this was to use business as a vehicle to help people in developing countries lift themselves out of poverty. We are creating opportunities, creating jobs, & providing access to capital. Creating an avenue to attract capital from outside the area and create investable assets that generate a profit, which, after delivering high returns to investors, can be reinvested into improving the living standards of the local indigenous community. Creating a private village development is the perfect starting point to do this.

But what if we also built a five-star hotel resort within the private gated community? This would create jobs for the local people, a viable investment opportunity for overseas investors, and attract people who want to buy into a gated community. A five-star luxury resort would bring high-spending tourists to the area.

Why stop there? To create a five-star resort, it needs an entire support ecosystem of different business types & skill sets. Building a hotel & private village needs all of the construction-related businesses. When complete, it impacts many other industries, from training providers to contractors, laundry companies, food providers & tourist attractions. The list is endless. In addition to investing in the hotel resort creation, what if we also invest in the entire supporting ecosystem, helping each business grow, develop, and deliver other contracts across the area?

To be clear, we invest in these assets, which attract capital from overseas. This model creates local employment, generates a profit, makes an excellent return to its investors, and the remaining investment returns pay for the community running costs, along with supporting the local indigenous community, building schools and healthcare facilities, providing food and water sources, which would otherwise be left to charity.

Creating this ecosystem creates a job & a good income source for each member of the indigenous local communities. It gives them an escape from poverty, meaning they no longer need handouts or charity to survive. This is about using our business experience to create opportunities for people, packaging those opportunities to attract overseas investment, & then using surplus profits to pay for the upkeep of the private community whilst also improving the living standards of the indigenous community.

We'll return to where we started this conversation around the circular economy concept. The only way our model works is to bring money from outside the community through investment. We do this by offering attractive investment opportunities in the private village community, the hotel resort, and the other local businesses. After the capital is in place, we must only use local companies that employ local people as much as possible. Ideally, this would focus on the local companies we've invested in.

In reality, this is the romantic version of the model. Still, in real life, we could never service 100% of our needs from our local ecosystem. For example, a five-star resort needs a five-star team of chefs to prepare the food. It's doubtful these could be sourced from within the indigenous local community.

Likewise, the hotel and other businesses might need to buy certain products or services externally to the ecosystem, such as consulting services or some manufactured products. These costs should be treated as investments, expecting to generate much higher returns than they cost. This is the actual circular economy. A real circular economy is one where everything stays inside the ecosystem & where it's made sustainable by design. This is true sustainability.

This model can be adapted and used at any scale—from your personal life to your business, local community, or country. While I've focused the model on the developing nations of Africa, it can also be used as an alternative system in developed nations.

My particular focus is on countries in the developing world because these possess a much better attitude towards opportunity on a logical level. On an emotional level, people in these countries trigger that emotional response inside my body, which I mentioned earlier.

As my previous stories demonstrated, businesses in the UK find excuses NOT to do things. However, I've found that people in developing nations tend to have a *'we'll find a way to do it'* attitude, much like myself.

Everything discussed in this chapter is based on a *'Profit-For-Purpose'* model. Profit-for-purpose is about creating a vehicle that can attract investment and using that investment to generate revenue and profit from a business venture. After repaying investors, surplus profits are reinvested into the *'purpose'*, investing them into other projects that drive toward the main objective. In our case, the aim is to lift the local communities out of extreme poverty.

I've received some hate online since I started talking about this model. Some say, *'You're opportunistically using cheap local labour to build five-star resorts so that you can make mega profits'*. Our model is rooted in the cause, & we created this model to try & alleviate that problem.

But to answer any critics who might think the same way. As I'm from the UK, you might imagine that if we didn't use local people to build a resort, we'd send people from the UK.

The problem with doing this, without considering the 30-day visa restrictions, would make the project financially unviable. It would cost more than the finished project was worth. We pay for flights, hotels, food, and 'work-away' pay rates. This would mean the project was never built.

For every resort we build, around £40 million filters through that local economy. If the project is a private village, that number is closer to £100 million. If we used UK staff & businesses to deliver the project, none of this investment would even touch that country's financial system.

By using our Profit-For-Purpose model, we're investing any future profits into the broader local ecosystem, we're investing in the supply chain, we're investing in schools, we're investing in the education system, we're investing in local food production, we're investing in creating localized water & energy generation, & in the longer term, we're creating thousands of jobs for the local people through this model. If a project is financially unviable, none of this would ever happen. Yes, the local labour rates in a developing country are far less than the UK's equivalent. However, those increased profits aren't returning to the UK; they're being reinvested into that local ecosystem. This model can also work in the developed world; we have to start thinking at a higher level of consciousness.

Employee ownership

A business is just a group of people with a shared objective. Why shouldn't those involved in that business own a stake in it? It doesn't matter what the company does; the outcome is always the same. Employees who own part of the business will always go that bit extra in serving the customer. They'll spend money as if it's coming from their pocket. They'll hold fellow staff accountable to a higher standard and always think of ways to improve things.

Suppose business owners want to know why they can't find reliable staff. In that case, they have yet to understand that people no longer want to work for someone else's benefit while they get paid the bare minimum.

Employee ownership doesn't need to mean you've got 67 staff barking orders and deciding how the business operates day-to-day. Nothing much has changed in that regard. The company's senior directors set the direction as expected. Still, instead of keeping operating performance private, the senior team acts in the interests of each shareholder.

Every year, the business can hold a meeting of all its shareholders, where they might ask for ideas, feedback, or initiatives to improve the business. These ideas are then implemented over the following twelve months.

Funding the share purchase can be a problem for people working low-paid roles in the business, because most don't have deep savings just sitting around.

Every employee must buy in rather than just being gifted the shares because this way, they know it's worth something. Instead of each staff member buying shares in a single purchase, you could perform a phased buy-in once or twice yearly. They might buy in by working a reduced salary for a fixed period, with the salary discount used to buy the shares. The employees don't need to own a large percentage of the business; the founding team & external investors need to maintain majority ownership, so employee shares might only be a collective pool of less than 25% of total equity.

While we've discussed the overall business model for creating a sustainable community, in the following chapters, we'll examine the functioning systems of that community to build a sustainable

model around them.

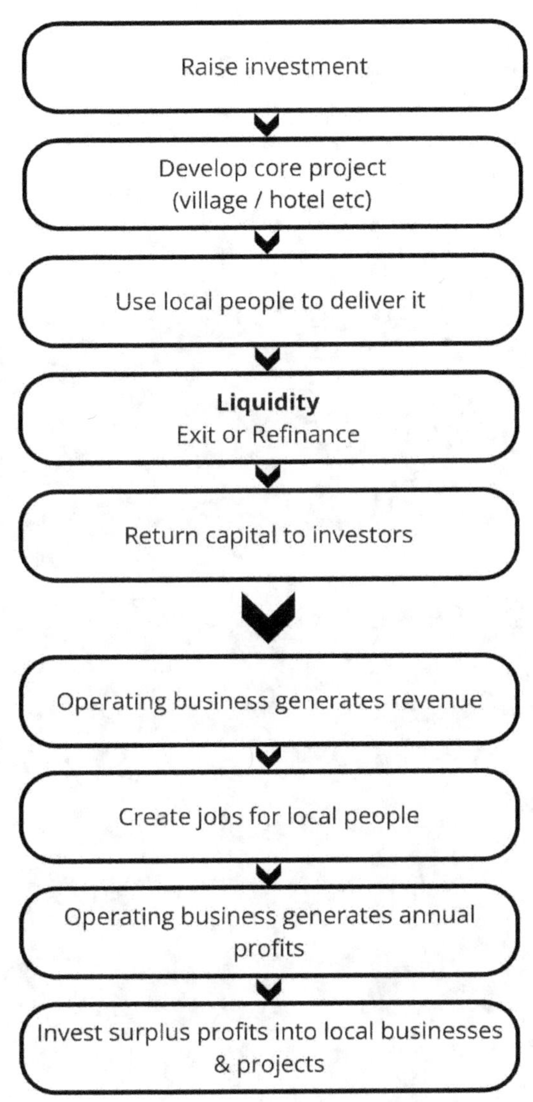

Raise investment
Develop core project
(village / hotel etc)
Use local people to deliver it
Liquidity
Exit or Refinance
Return capital to investors
Operating business generates revenue
Create jobs for local people
Operating business generates annual
profits
Invest surplus profits into local businesses
& projects

Root

In this chapter, we'll examine the foundations of every society and what we need to redesign a system that benefits the people.

Access to opportunity

If we look at the most deprived areas, we see the same effect, regardless of where we are. If you don't provide access to opportunities, people turn to other things that become a detriment to society.

Growing up in rural Scotland in the 90's, I left school two months before my 16th birthday. My classmates generally followed the same path that happens in most deprived areas. A small percentage, maybe 10%, attended university & left the area. 30% went down the apprenticeship route, and about 30% took an unskilled job. The rest were unemployed. This section of people just sat at home all day; some got into drugs, but many got into crime. In our area, the crime vacuum got swallowed up by drug trafficking. We lived about two hours from the nearest city & people were *'sold'* on the idea of improving their position in life by moving drugs from the city & bringing them into the rural communities.

Had these people been given access to opportunity, opportunities that would earn them equivalent levels of lifestyle or status as the drugs, how many people do you think would choose the crime route?

The problems in our society today stem from a lack of opportunities. All the significant opportunities in the world are often reserved for those who either went to an elite university or those from an aristocratic lineage. For example, suppose a child wants to compete in the Olympics. In that case, they'll encounter many obstacles to that selection shortlist. Even the best athlete must be *'approved'* to attend the event.

One of those first obstacles is knowing how to get into that field. Where would I start if I dreamt of making it to the 100-meter Olympic sprint? Then comes the lack of resources & the money to support such a journey. If you follow the story of Michael Edwards, better known as *'Eddie the Eagle'*, a British ski jumper from the 80s, coming from a typical working-class family, his dad a plasterer, his mum a housewife, he was seen as an embarrassment to the establishment, which meant they changed the rules, in an attempt to prevent him competing.

Even when he made it to the Olympics, he was mocked and made to look like an idiot on TV by the sporting media, probably hoping he'd just quietly go away if they put much media pressure on him and his family. Whilst the British establishment perceived him as an embarrassment, just the fact he persevered in chasing his dream AND reached the Olympics should be something for the British public to be proud of, & inspired by, but that was never the case. At best, he was seen by most of the British public as a disappointment.

It's the same in any field. In the corporate world, I've seen many boards of directors, & senior management teams being run by people who were *'parachuted'* into these positions, coming from a *'well-known'* family, or their father being a *'Lord'*. It's run by the *'old boys network'*, the old guard, & as they say, *'it's a big club and you ain't in it'*. The glass ceiling is real; it doesn't matter how hard you work; those positions are already reserved.

We have to start by opening up opportunities to people. We have to move into an 'opportunity mindset'. That means sharing and collaboration. Rather than trying to do everything ourselves, we should look around and ask, who might be suitable to do this with me?

Imagine, for a second, a secluded island in the middle of the ocean. Let's say we've built a hotel on the island, and with all the paying guests, we've generated this massive pile of laundry every day. But we notice the neighbouring peninsula also has an enormous pile of laundry. Currently, we do all this laundry ourselves. Here's where the opportunity mindset comes in.

Instead of doing it all ourselves, we ask, *'Who might be looking for an opportunity?'* Why don't we set up a business to wash this dirty laundry with those people? Suppose there's a small group of people.

In that case, it means we solve our problem whilst also giving each individual an opportunity to improve their status & position in life.

These individuals need to gain business experience, so why don't we mentor them and keep them on track with the business? Bringing several motivated individuals together under the same company solves the problem of reliance on one person. We could find an experienced business operator and parachute them into running the business until the rest are experienced enough to run it themselves. That would also protect the investment needed to set it up.

Access to capital

A similar story applies to Formula One. Thousands of kids globally have grown up competing in kart racing. But it takes so much money, plus having the right connections to get you into the next level of the sport.

I'm not ruling out hard work, but you can be the fastest on the track; if you don't have two pennies to rub together, you may as well forget it. Having competed in rallying, I witnessed this situation with many people I raced against. Most are just priced out of the sport. When I competed, I had no ambitions of being a world champion; it had been my schoolboy dream to compete, so living it out was enough to satisfy my desires. Still, I also realized that the person with the *'biggest bank account'* won.

Over five years, I invested my entire salary into building a car & then competing. To compete at the front of the field at the national level, I've heard of privateer competitors that can spend a million pounds in one season. To compete at the world championship level, driving with the manufacturer teams means having a budget of about four million pounds to cover a single season, & that's without considering the cost of significant car damage throughout the season.

Most who compete at these levels own huge, well-known businesses that pay for their hobby, or they come from famous families with historic success in the sport & so sponsors are willing to back them based on their surname.

Along with providing access to opportunity, the next objective is to provide access to capital, helping to deliver these opportunities. This doesn't mean giving capital to anyone wishing to compete in Formula One motorsport; I use this only as an example. They are instead creating a ladder whereby anyone can access the funds needed by creating revenue-generating projects, & funding their lifestyle from the rewards of that project. This can be done by attracting investment from outside of the local economy. Alternatively, community members can pool their capital to keep the cycle going. Every time an investment succeeds, it feeds into the system to help others in the community.

Community investment fund

If we look at small businesses, less than 1% of investment dollars make it to this part of the economy. For the rest, a lucky few receive investment via *'ordinary people'* collectively pooling their savings and investing through various platforms. Look at any crowdfunding platform; probably less than twenty businesses seek investment there. When you consider there are six million small businesses in the UK, you can see how small this pool of alternative funding is.

The business *'startup'* space is equally dyer. Unless you're a tech startup with a track record of scaling multiple tech startups, the possibility of receiving investment from the investment community is ZERO. Such startups rely on money from friends, family, or personal savings.

The problem with investing in these types of opportunities at this current time is that 50% of businesses fail in their first year. 90% fail within five years. Only 4% make it to 10 years.

The criteria for investing into a business are:
1. It has to be established with a strong customer demand
2. A complete management team must be in place to run the business.

Without these two factors, there's a solid chance you'll lose your money. The reason is that most people starting a business have never done it before. They're navigating a path blindfolded, with no compass, no map, no torch, but lots of cliff edges.

As a business grows and gets more customers, it faces other problems, like dealing with staff issues, managing cash flow, and balancing customer demand with the capacity to deliver. All of this is new to most startups, & there needs to be more help, training or support for these businesses to access this information. The system isn't weighted in their favour.

When they've reached the stage of employing a management team, they've typically learnt how to overcome these issues and hopefully have experts managing each area of the business. The other risk with investing in owner-managed small companies and startups is that something could happen to the business owner, meaning they can't work for six months. Without people to take over in their absence, the business is dead, and any investment dies with it.

With an opportunity fund, we also need sound risk management to reduce the impact of any investments failing. This means having strong people to manage each opportunity, business, or investment.

More importantly, companies need proper direction, guidance, and a shared ethos of creating opportunities for others in the community as part of their day-to-day operating model. Each business within the investment portfolio should share our ethos and model of supporting a local supply chain.

There needs to be a method for returning & recycling the investment back into the central pot, so that it can be reinvested into more opportunities as fast as possible.

A family office is a team that manages an individual's wealth. They invest capital into various categories of investment, whether property, shares, precious metals, or business. The family office structure intends to make investments that provide a return on that investment, grow the central pot value, and provide the beneficiary with an income large enough to cover their living expenses & costs.

Using the same principles of a family office, we invest that capital into what we call *'value creation'* infrastructure. This means investing it into buildings & businesses that will generate revenue, & make an ongoing return on that investment. This investment fund could be expanded to generate sufficient income to continuously grow the community infrastructure over time, paid for by the yearly returns.

Supporting local

What opportunities could you offer to people in the local community? Suppose you're currently buying from large national or international companies. How might you shift that to buy from local businesses instead? What would need to happen for that to become your *'go-to'* operating process?

The more we create and support local businesses, the more opportunities will be made for local people. This cycle grows bigger the more we do it.

Few have considered this idea, but how successful would a business be if its customers invested in it, too? Customers who invest in their supply chain should be customers for life. The traditional procurement process for businesses is one of the least efficient and time-wasting processes I've ever encountered.

If a customer invests in your business, it would remove the need to compete against eight other firms, with only one supplier winning a contract, whilst the other seven waste their time. If a business wins one contract in every five it tenders, that's an 80% saving on our time & energy. In other words, if you only tendered for the contracts you would win, that means you'd only work on a Monday, & then spend the rest of the week doing something productive. If a customer owns its supply chain, it's motivated to help them develop. Rather than bidding for individual contracts, the conversation moves to pitching for investment from clients. That's one conversation, one pitch, & then focus on delivering what they need.

The vulnerable

There will always be some people in our society who need support, whether it be a safety net if they have a failed business, for example, or someone who can't support themselves due to old age, disability, or perhaps even being orphaned at a young age.

In the Formula chapter, we've examined a model for generating income through investment vehicles. Still, now that we understand this concept, we need to ask ourselves whether this might be a solution to support the community's needs and pay for those costs. Rather than just paying for the costs to help the vulnerable, this could be a route to paying *everyone's* living expenses across the entire community.

To take it one step further, if we have no living expenses, then we have nothing forcing us to work in jobs we don't like.

We can each do what interests us most, & what's best for the whole community. People who enjoy growing food can focus on growing food for the community. The person that likes teaching can work in the school. You get the idea. The artists of the community can create great pieces of art, & sell them to the outside world to bring in more income revenue to the community.

One thing we've not looked at yet is the people who receive support from the system, for example, those who can't work to earn money, or they've fallen off their path in some way & those who are disabled. How does our model work for them? This all comes back to designing it for the new model. Everything you witness with the current system is just the effect of multiple knee-jerk reactions by the government. A sustainable system shouldn't need knee-jerk responses because it's proactively designed from day one.

Now, we need to answer the question of what happens to the vulnerable in our society.

These individuals need specific resources, whether food, energy, shelter, or something more specific, like equipment or support from a carer. As with the rest of our community, this resource demand is designed for in the system from day one.

Suppose resources need to be purchased from outside of the community. In that case, the model is designed to generate additional revenues it needs so that these resources can be purchased externally.

We've talked about living in a *money-less* economy, having your resources generated within the confines of that community space. This model works; everyone receives everything they need. But to purchase any external resources we need, we have to generate sufficient income from the external world, & we do that by making additional investments into revenue-generating assets.

Development

Considering that we live on an isolated island in the middle of the ocean, how will we pay for the construction of all the infrastructure, the buildings, and the basic development of the island? Of course, this doesn't include the cost of the land itself.

Phase one involves performing an inventory of the land to identify what resources we have available. What needs upgrading, repair, or improvement, and what will we need to bring in from the outside world? This is where the initial costs lie.

After we have an inventory of the site, phase two considers any value-creation opportunities. What can we do that will maximize revenue-generating opportunities from the outside world? When we've created a development plan, we should consider what infrastructure the development plan will need.

What buildings are required? How many people? What skill sets? How will we feed everyone? How will we house them? How will we manage waste from all these activities? Will we have a water supply large enough to feed all our requirements? & How much space is needed to accommodate everything?

Phase three is the build phase, which could be delivered under its sequencing. We are starting small, building the bare minimum & scaling it up as those value-creation activities are picking up pace. We don't want to build infrastructure, hotels & homes to house 1,000 people if we only need three houses on day one. Having a more minor development that can be scaled up and expanded easily is a better option & requires less financial & physical resources to bring the idea to life.

When considering how to pay for phase one, there are a few options that could be considered as follows:

License to occupy: A license to occupy is generally used in locations where it's illegal for a foreign entity to own the land. The occupants gain a land permit, similar to a long-term lease. The license is typically a 50-year renewable license, with a further 50-year extension. The amount paid is comparable to basic ground rent in Western countries.

Land purchase: An outright purchase of the land is a route used less often now unless the intention is to divide the land into individual parcels, develop them, and sell them immediately.

Landowner equity investment: The landowner is an equity investor, providing the land rather than capital to the project. This means they receive a portion of all revenue and sale proceeds from the completed project.

Land donation: With land donation the landowner donates the land to the project at no cost. This is generally done from a philanthropic perspective or where the local community will benefit from the project. This may depend on the project vehicle's jurisdiction and legal structure. Often, this happens when the government donates the land to a project to be developed for the local community's use or betterment, for example, by donating land to build a new energy plant to which the local community will have access.

Other options may include:

Pooling of capital: A group of people pool their capital to be part of the community later on.

Skills exchange: If someone wants to be part of a project but needs capital, they could invest their time & skills in exchange for equity in the project. This can work for any role within the project, whether it is someone with a vast network of investors, who might be paid based on every successful introduction, or if it's someone that is a qualified plumber providing the plumbing services to the project & they're paid in equity in the project. This equity stake can later be exchanged for equity in the community or receive a share of any future profits from the project, precisely as an investor will do.

Tokenization: Similar to some of the ideas already discussed, if a person provides something of value to the project or the completed community, such as growing food and selling it to the community, they can be paid using a token system. These tokens can then be exchanged within the community, either for a house or for someone else's services within the same community. This is the start of a new localized monetary system.

Society

Imagine a society where everyone was equal & there was no class system. There would be no reason for anyone to burden themselves with debt, attempting to portray a false image of wealth.

Attending any school reunion, you'll witness a *'dick swinging contest'* where people pretend their chipolata is a frankfurter, trying to portray how much more successful they've become over their former classmates.

It doesn't matter at which end of the social spectrum you look. Go to Monaco Marina, and you'll notice everyone competing against each other for who has the biggest yacht, apparently as a sign of who is the most successful. Whilst Jimmy has a 50-meter superyacht, believing he's the *'big dawg of Dagenham'*, when he goes to Monaco, he's looked down on as being *'one of the peasants'* by the guy with the 200-meter megayacht.

Watch the school run. In some areas, you'll notice all the mums trying to outcompete each other with their 4x4 SUVs, who's the most expensive, who's the biggest. Whose is the newest?
Imagine that, growing up, girls aren't interested in cars, but when it's about outshining their peers

from the playground in later life, they take a keen interest in them.

This is the type of society we live in today. It's all an inner desire for others to see us as having higher social status. On a subconscious level, we need to be recognized and validated by other people.

Of course, the mental health crisis prevalent in society today is just one of the many effects of how our society operates. Depression and suicide are all fueled by people living these pretend lifestyles, & even they, when they come to terms with & realize their life isn't how they'd hoped it would be.

This comes back to how someone views their position in life. If you view life as a scorecard, where the person with the most material possessions wins, then 99% of people will always be unhappy with that picture.

There's always something else to buy or something that someone else owns. You'll need an endless supply of money to play that game.

Instead, what if we viewed our position in life as whether we enjoy our daily life experience? Do we have time with our family? Do we have meaningful connections with our friends, work colleagues, and business connections? How do we make an impact, however small, on each of these human connections?

If we remove the need for material possessions, and everyone has everything they need and want, suddenly, life becomes about more than just having that latest status symbol on our wrist.

Moving away from trying to outclimb your social circle and having people admire you is the only way we move away from the perception of a class-based system.

As we know it today, the class system breaks down society. Ultimately, the class system was created by the ruling class, those you might worship as *'the royals'*; without both the ruling class & the peasant class, they'd be seen as equals, so our ancestors would never have paid them any attention. It also creates this demand for debt, as we use it as a ladder to climb the ladder of wealth perception.

Elders

In our current system, people go to work & then retire. At this point, they either die within a few months or spend their retirement doing anything to keep themselves busy. Alternatively, they'll sit watching daytime TV or old war films. This was how my Grandad lived for 20 years after he retired. After building his house, & going on the occasional holiday, or doing the odd garden project, the rest of the time was spent watching old war films. It's like a person loses their purpose when they retire.

Imagine an alternative retirement. Rather than leaving the workplace, we use it to pass on all that valuable life experience, & help the next generation. The education system is a joke, but with a revolution in how we learn, we can all become a mentor or guides to those who come after us. If you're a retired 70-year-old, your value is no longer in *'doing the work'*; it is in sharing the experiences you endured & passing them on to others. What if you could shape a younger person's life so they don't make those same mistakes?

Think about all the mistakes you've made in your life and all the lessons you've learned from them. How can the human race evolve if those lessons aren't passed on to younger generations? Otherwise, it becomes a repeating cycle where each generation never evolves, going through the same experience but starting from zero each time.

In ancient traditions across many cultures, we had *'elders'*; these were the wise men of the community who'd lived many experiences. These elders passed on their life wisdom to the rest of the community, preventing them from making bad decisions. For instance, if a mistake such as going to war were made without the elders' wise counsel, an inexperienced leader might overreact, and the whole community might be slaughtered.

We can have modern-day *'elders'*, each with experience in different fields. It starts with school-age children learning about particular subjects, much like we have the technical apprenticeship model we use now.

Rather than the need for *'qualified teachers'*, we have someone who's worked a role in that subject across many decades & can pass on those real-life lessons, & shortcuts, a traditional *'teacher'* doesn't know about.

This doesn't mean an end to teachers; teachers know how to help someone learn. The teachers aren't the problem in the education system; the problem is what they're forced to teach & how.

After school age comes mentoring for people who want to start a business, these elders combine their experiences while working to a framework for starting a business. These elders can guide and assist in the day-to-day running of those businesses. Then, as the company grows, it needs more of a board-level guide, people who have already walked that path.

Guidance can cover all areas, not just business or education. There's a need for guidance in social skills, connection, communication, roblem-solving, specialist skills like growing food or emergency healthcare, understanding who you are and your purpose here, and even relationships.

This is what's currently missing in our system. Look at the most searched topics on YouTube, and you'll notice people searching for foundational-level knowledge, like *'how to have a relationship'*. With data like this, we have a clear gap in our education, and we need to learn these subjects as an integral part of our early-stage development. There's a profound detachment from our foundational needs in favour of filling our lives with needless information and technology.

In addition to supporting society, the elders model provides older people with a sense of purpose.

Education

What if the education system had a stake in the outcome of your life? Rather than trying to fill seats, it could focus on the specific knowledge you need to learn to achieve what you want. How would this work in practice, though?

Rather than you paying for the education either directly or indirectly, the education provider would fund it. Instead of learning the intricate details of every subject, you'd identify what the outcome was, & the provider would teach you the specific topics you needed to learn to achieve that outcome. Instead of wasting five years learning a subject, it might only take a few months. From that point, the provider would receive a share of your future earnings from that learning, up to a predetermined amount, similar to an investor funding a project in a joint venture with you. The provider is aligned with you & what you want to achieve, so they're also motivated to provide the support you need to reach that goal.

Conclusion

We called this chapter the Root. Everything we've discussed is the foundation of everything in society. The reason we have crime, homelessness or drug epidemics is because the foundations of our society are broken. The natural answer that people point to is that socialism will fix our societal problems. Socialism means giving more power to governments but it was the governments that created this problem. Socialism is not the solution. We can only fix these problems by focusing on our society's very foundations and getting those correct. That's when things change. Fix the Root, and the flower will bloom, but without the strong Root, there is no flower.

Exchange

In this chapter, we will look at the principle of how we exchange value, moving away from a corrupt monetary system controlled by people who don't work for the people's highest and best interests.

Economy

The Oxford Dictionary defines an *'economy'* or to *'economize'* as cutting back our spending. This is an *'economy'* mindset.

If we cut back our spending, there's less money circulating in the system, leading to poverty, poor health, crime & numerous other problems we can see today. The current *'economy'* based system is the root of most issues we have in society, and the way to fix these issues is to increase money circulation in the system. Please note that when I say 'increase money circulation', I do not mean to increase money supply, otherwise known in recent times as *'quantitive easing'* or *'money printing'*.

When we say *'we want a growth economy'*, it's like saying, *'we want growth constraints'*, it's like saying, *'I want a warm ice cream'*, yet we've been programmed in a way to believe this is how things should be—a world of constraints. Nature doesn't exist in a world of constraints. Nature creates more than enough for everything to flourish.

Have you ever questioned why the universe doesn't prevent the nettles from growing or those bramble bushes that grow out of control every summer?

No, because it's just nature. The birds & the bees have more than enough food to live *'an abundant life'*; they don't live a frugal or constrained existence. So why do 99% of humans believe this is how we should live?

There are enough resources & land on this planet for everyone to have what they need. We don't have a resource problem; we have a fair distribution problem.

I remember when I was a child, I'd always wonder why things didn't make sense. As children, we instinctively know when something's not right, but like me, we're told by society to *'get on with it'* and *'don't ask questions'*. Those spotlighting anything wrong with the world get punished by their family, the education system, or society.

So, if we can't call it an economy, what can we call it? Use whichever terms you want, but I will call it *'money circulation'*. While there might be better labels, I hope you can identify with my topic. In a future fairer society, we call it *'value circulation'* or *'value flow'*.

According to the dictionary, the opposite of *'economy'* is *'to be wasteful'*. Again, even this was twisted somewhere along the way. It's like saying that if we have abundant money circulation, it's wasteful. Nature doesn't waste anything. Nature thrives. I can only imagine that those who control the current system of scarcity need the population to believe this is the only way for humans to function, either cutting back or being wasteful.

Taxation

If you work for a week, & you get paid £1,000 for doing that work. At the end of every week, Tony, the local gangster, comes to your house & takes £500 for himself.

If you ever try to avoid paying him the money, he'll hunt you down & throw you in a cage.

If this were the case, you wouldn't be happy, yet we quietly accept it when that mobster organization we call *'government'* does the same thing. Taxation is theft. Taxation is slavery. We do all the hard work on Mr Jones's plantation, but Mr Jones reap most of the fruits from our labour despite never doing anything to earn it. In most countries, the government's share is more than 50% in direct & indirect taxes. Suppose you're a small business owner in the UK. Did you know that to extract profits from your company and put it in your pocket? In that case, you pay 63% of those original profits in tax?

We'll work Monday & Tuesday for ourselves, but we work Wednesday, Thursday & Friday for the government.

The direct tax on our salaries is just at the surface level. Taxation is on everything we buy, even the food we buy in supermarkets. While some countries don't charge sales tax or VAT on food at the checkout, it's already built into the sale price. Import taxes, transport taxes, retail space taxes, etc., all have direct or indirect taxes built into them. Unless you're growing it all yourself, you're being taxed on it.

It gets worse than that. Still, a company creates an unbelievable amount of tax for the government, in indirect & direct taxes. A business is like a slot machine that pays out on every spin to the government, whether you make a profit or not. The direct taxes are apparent. They're the ones you'll already be conscious of - corporation tax, capital gains tax, national insurance or social security.

Every business you engage with either adds taxes directly or builds them into their costs, the indirect taxes they've had to pay to deliver what you buy.

Did you know that over 80% of the price you pay for fuel in your car is tax? How do you feel when you realize you've just spent £100 to fill your car with fuel, but the actual value was only £20?

Compare the cost of red diesel. At the current price comparison, in the UK this week, the cost per litre of red diesel is 52 pence per litre. Compared to regular diesel, which is £2.00 per litre. Farmers use red diesel, but the only difference is how much tax the government collects on each option. Risk getting caught using red diesel in your vehicle, & the *'crime'* carries a heavy fine and a potential prison sentence. The only reason it carries such a heavy penalty is because a bunch of scammers need to intimidate you into compliance.

We haven't even considered the death, wealth, & property taxes that we all have to pay.

But what about all the tax you generate as a bi-product of operating your business? First, you've got VAT or sales tax. Then you've got the sales tax you pay to your suppliers. Staff taxes: each of your staff pays tax & social security. Your supply chain also has staff that each pay tax & social security. They, too, have their supply chain, each paying VAT, Staff taxes, corporation tax, capital gains tax, dividend tax, etc. You buy vehicles with taxes on them, import duty, fuel taxes, company car taxes, and benefit-in-kind taxes. I don't wish to bore you with the line-by-line details, so I'll summarize them as best I can.

I'll give you an example to make it easier to understand. Let's take an average small business; for easy calculation, let's say it has £1 million in sales revenue, though the actual figure doesn't matter. This average small business generates around £800,000 in direct & indirect taxes for the government annually. That's right, you generate around 80% of your total revenue in direct & indirect taxes.

The average small business makes a 10% bottom-line net profit, while the government makes 80%. If you're a small business owner, you've got to question, who exactly are you doing this for?

I understand this is quite complex for the average *'non-financial'* person. Still, if you own a small business, you'll recognize some of those figures I've mentioned.

Don't tell me the government supports you as a small business owner. *'Oh, but Wayne, they gave me financial help through Covid'*. No, what they did was ensure your compliance with staying at home. What they did was guarantee they'd continue to keep getting paid themselves. Oh, & by the way, that wasn't *'Free money'*. That furlough money is paid for by increasing everyone's taxation rates. Those COVID loans, which just loaded your business with debt it can't afford, run at 8% above the base rate, but guess who controls that base rate? That's right, THEY do !!!

But if they had not set up these *'facilities'*, nobody would stay at home, as without an income stream in this artificial system, nobody survives - and *noncompliance doesn't serve the*ir interests.

You might ask, *'If nobody paid taxes, how would we care for the vulnerable in our society? And, how do we pay for the bins to be emptied?'*

The first thing I want to clarify is about tax-free countries. How do they pay for all their needs? Tax-free countries are often also the wealthiest countries, yet how could that be if the government's income source doesn't come from taxation?

To the conventional mind, it isn't easy to comprehend, especially after so much socialist brainwashing over the last few decades.

These countries offer programs to incentivize and entice wealthy families and businesses to base themselves in the country. Wealthy families spend lots of money, and companies create jobs and investments, which, in both cases, increases the flow of money in that country's economy.

Remember, this is what we discussed at the start of the chapter: increasing money flow reduces poverty.

If there's more money flowing, & it's not being taken off the table by the government, naturally, every *player* in the game has more money flowing through them. After everyone has more money flowing through them, these countries' second strategy is a *pay for what you use* model. In other words, if you want your bins emptied, you pay for it. But if you have no bins, you don't pay for it.

The same applies to every area of life, education, healthcare, etc. That's fine if you're wealthy, but what about everyone else, and how does this work in practice? Well, imagine how things work in a regular *'high tax'* country. Your bins are collected & paid for by the government - with your money. The government is acting on your behalf as a purchasing agent.

The problem is governments are very inefficient. In some countries, some of that money pays for corruption; in others, it just gets swallowed up with red tape, duplication, and general bullshit. I know this because I've spent my career supplying services to government departments, & I know exactly how they operate.

In our companies, we could bid against the government's own Direct Labour Organisation (their in-house team); our bid would be half the price of theirs, & we'd still make a good profit.

If the government had been efficient, it would've been impossible for us to do that, especially considering our staff were travelling daily to their location, staying in hotels, etc. In contrast, their staff are already based in that location.

Now, if you go out to the local waste collection company, & request they empty your bins, it'll be expensive. They've got to send a truck with two staff, it could be a 20-mile round trip, they've got to dispose of that rubbish, & they've got to recycle the rest. That might cost, for example, £300 to you as an individual. But £295 of that cost will probably be made up of indirect expenses, like travel time, the price of the truck, the two staff, etc.

But if you teamed up with all your neighbours and formed a bulk buying cooperative responsible for all shared services, the cost might be reduced to, say, £2 each because all that indirect cost is shared between 2,000 buyers instead of just one.

Buying anything in bulk means you can access a more significant discount than buying as an individual.

To understand the problem with taxes, we first must understand how most countries function. The common misunderstanding is that our taxes pay for things like the welfare system, the police, the healthcare system, our roads, our transport system, etc.

This lie has been spread to keep you ignorant. If people knew their taxes weren't paying for nurses, police, & teachers, many would stop paying their taxes altogether.

We live in a debt-based financial system. This is why we get recessions predictably every fifteen years or so - just like clockwork. A recession happens because money has been taken out of circulation. That money is debt.

Who controls debt? The central banks do. We're told that recessions happen due to some *'black swan'* event. When you realize it's the same people that control the debt supply, to those who own the swans, you start to see that nothing happens by coincidence.

Central banks are not governments. Central banks are private corporations that lend money to governments. When you pay taxes, those taxes pay for the *interest* on the debts borrowed in a previous period. But those debts have compounded interest over many decades.

Did you know the UK has only just finished paying for the debt it borrowed during World War II?

Would you think it is a coincidence that central banks finance many wars worldwide, too? That's correct; they finance the warmongers, and then they finance the rebuilding of the country after it's been obliterated. You might say it's in their interest to make these wars happen. It's a very twisted, sick little game; and we're all paying for it.

So, if we're only paying for the previous debt pile, how do nurses, teachers, police, and infrastructure get paid for? Simple: the government takes on MORE DEBT. The government borrows more money, increasing the interest that we, the people, have to pay. It's a model that isn't sustainable; eventually, the system implodes.

A better alternative to this current system is to remove taxation altogether. If you've ever played Monopoly, imagine every time you 'pass go', but rather than collecting £200, you paid £200 instead. Every time you pass Go, the banker takes £200 out of circulation in the game. The game wouldn't last very long. Taking money out of the game prevents anyone from *investing*. The less invested, the weaker and less wealthy everyone is within that society.

It's the same with our government tax system. Every time we pay taxes, we reduce the amount of money circulating in the system. When the average person has spare cash, they buy something with it, go on holiday, buy a training course, or invest it in an asset. It keeps circulating. A system that removes money from the game isn't good for the people within that game.

If you're unfortunate enough to live in a country that extorts its citizens, it's hard to implement an alternative solution, without being thrown in a prison cell. This book is more like a bridge between this tyrannical dystopia we're living in at the moment and the future vision of rebuilding society in the utopian future we all need. I hope you choose one with zero taxation if you choose a country to host your new community project or expand your business.

But in the interim, we can consider these ideas and use legal ways to reduce the tax we pay so that more of it stays in our local circulation system.

Rewarding value creation

In this section, we will discuss two concepts relating to a different way of thinking about how money flows in the local system and how we might support those who cannot help themselves.

In our island example, getting everything we need as a community from one island is impossible. We need to buy supplies from outside that community, so we need something to exchange.

While nobody would be doing *'work'* in the traditional sense of *'needing to work'*, opportunities still need investing. The labour pool would be reorganized, with people being magnetized toward activities they prefer doing.

In this system, there's less emphasis on people being paid in the traditional sense. Instead, there might be more opportunities seeking investment as each person moves onto their true path in life.

The future of society is a future without money. It may take a century to reach that point. Still, if you imagine, money is just a bunch of numbers on a screen, and it doesn't exist anyway. In its current form, it's a human-created construct. And actually, it's a limiting factor preventing us from moving forward. Think about that training course you want to attend, which costs £10,000. If you can scrape that money together, that course might change your life; you might learn information that impacts 1000 other people's lives. You might meet your future husband or wife on that course, & have four kids together. The problem is, if you're unemployed, & have no money, it'll never happen, & so nothing moves forward. If that course didn't cost anything, because money didn't exist, everyone would have access to their true life path.

There's an argument that says we don't value what's free. That's true, but only in the current paradigm. See, if everything were free, you'd only resonate with the things indeed for you. If someone gives you a free book or a free course if that subject resonates with you & if you are interested in it, it wouldn't matter what the cost was; you'd participate because you're interested in it. Nobody would ever use their local library if this weren't the case.

We don't value what's free in the current paradigm because we get sold on other people's paths. What I mean by this is you see someone who got rich from day trading shares, you notice what a fantastic lifestyle they're living, you see how they've had a movie produced, documenting their life, and now they're famous. So you decide, that's what you want to do. The idea of trading shares in your own life never entered your mind until you watched a movie about that individual.

This is how brainwashing works. It's also why 99% of the population is chasing a life path never meant for them. When that training course is offered for free, it loses its perceived value because you never really wanted it to start. If it were your true life path, the price wouldn't matter if you could afford it.

Chasing someone else's path boils down to chasing something on a subconscious level. You're chasing money, status, or love - your subconscious believes you lack love or recognition, so we chase these things to fill a hole. This all works below the surface, but we tell ourselves stories to justify it on a conscious awareness level.

Take the property industry as an example. In the last two decades, the UK property industry has been flooded with people becoming property developers, investors, and trainers. For most, the reason behind doing it is to *get money*. They're chasing money.

If you gave them a choice between sitting on a beach or managing tenants, which would they choose?

If you take the money away, most people will resonate with what they're called to do rather than chase money. If the trainers provided that training for free, we'd see a rapid shift away from that path and into something else.

We're often told that money is just an exchange for the value we've provided to someone. If this were true, how much value would you place on a disabled person being able to shower themselves? Nobody wants to sit in their own urine for weeks at a time, do they? The nurse doing this job would surely be a billionaire if this value exchange concept were genuine. Instead, we live in a world where a banker receives a bonus equivalent to ten years' wages for that nurse. Did the banker provide more value than the nurse?

Imagine a world where people are rewarded for the value they create for society. A place where instead of having a Sunday Times Rich List, we have a 'value creation list, people that might still be very wealthy, but all the wealth was created by helping to improve society rather than detracting from it. What if those who detracted from our society, those who make large businesses off the back of causing massive gambling, alcohol or drug addiction, rather than being some of the wealthiest people on the planet from their ill-gotten gains, instead were jailed? If this were the case, we could flip the current society on its head, & we'd see every carer in the country driving high-performance supercars to work. In our freedom framework, people are rewarded for value creation.

What is most valuable to that community? What is most valuable to neighbouring communities? This is how a genuine free market society should function.

Energize

This chapter examines how we can finance our Profit-For-Purpose project, whether a private community, a resort development, or some other business venture. We'll also discuss how to create an attractive investment opportunity and the fundamentals of the investment vehicle.

For over 13 years, I've received pitches from people looking for investment. Through this process, I've noticed some common themes across more than 1,000 different opportunities that I've looked at.

During this time, I've also built my network with over 18,000 professional and institutional level investors, so I understand what makes an attractive investment opportunity to an experienced investor, and it's probably different from what you think.

In this chapter, I will present you with the fundamentals of a viable investment opportunity. Without attracting external investment into our model, the whole thing will never happen. Whilst we'll use the example of raising money for a hotel resort, the same principles can be applied to any business or project.

Trading history

Investment capital is generally thin on the ground when investing in the developing world. The perception of corruption, crime, & a general lack of transparency are all factors that make it increasingly more complex to raise investment for projects.

So, rather than raising money for a new startup idea, I'm only considering raising investment for a business with an established trading history. With an established company, the investment process will be more straightforward. The larger & more established a business is, the process becomes more effortless still.

If the project is in a frontier market country, we must make it as low-risk & attractive as possible. About 95% of investment capital goes to 'mid-market' or larger-sized investments. So unless you've got a business with £20m in profits, you're targeting the much smaller pools of capital. For the hotel resort in our model, whilst the resort will be new, or at least renovated & upgraded, the resort's management will need to be an established hotel operator. The business is a five-star spa resort, so the hotel operator must also operate an existing five-star resort elsewhere. There are two main reasons for this. First, they know what a guest experience should look like and what the guest expects of their time at the resort.

Secondly, as a trading business, they'll already have a database of happy past guests to whom they can sell a new location. Guests who are comfortable spending at the level a five-star resort demands.

Theme

While we will discuss *'Theme'* in the context of a hotel to explain this concept, the same applies to any business. The theme concerns knowing your customers, their expected experience, and how you position the offering in the market. Let's look at an example.

Every mainstream hotel chain has a theme. It might be roadside motels, conference hotels, airport hotels, or something more specialist. When you see a hotel struggling, it doesn't have a theme. It needs to find out who it is, its customers, and what those customers need. It's not enough to be a four-star hotel. The grading is just an indication of the furnishing level; it's not a theme.

Without a theme, the business competes against the whole market. An airport hotel offers a very different experience than an adult-only beach resort. The guests' requirements and price expectations are very different. Having a theme reduces your competition from the entire market to just competing with a handful of similar businesses.

Basing your business on a theme means identifying precisely who your customers are, what type of offering they need, and what price they're willing to pay. It also lets you identify your competitors in the market so you can position your business and differentiate from them.

Brand

The next thing for a hotel resort is to have a legacy brand above the door. When I talk about legacy brands, I mean a brand known among the target customers, regardless of location.

Legacy brands are the iconic brands known far & wide, such as *Six Senses*, *Four Seasons*, and *Marriott*, all known and respected for the service they provide guests within that five-star experience. Regular hotel brands of more traditional local or regional hotel groups aren't as well recognized by the public; they don't have the brand recognition required to attract new customers.

A brand is more than just a logo. It is how customers perceive your business, driven by their experience dealing with it. The logo is a small part of how a customer identifies the brand. A regional or local hotel brand generally only applies to local or regional customers. A hotel investor usually likes a hotel investment to be branded by one of the legacy brands because it attracts a higher level of valuation in the market.

Legacy brands have invested millions of dollars into campaigns to raise brand awareness & improve their brand recognition, not just with past guests but also to attract guests from other legacy brands. Legacy brands don't necessarily have to be global; some focus initially on a particular continent but generally intend to expand that reach to a worldwide awareness over time.

Owning a legacy brand, you need to have brand recognition, if not globally, certainly be well established on the continents where you have a presence. Regarding location numbers, a legacy brand needs to offer a variety of locations, with the same product style being offered in all places, regardless of country or continent.

Brand recognition with investment in PR campaigns can be achieved when you reach ten or more locations on one continent. One example is the *Rocco Forte Hotel group*, a 5-star hotel group mainly focused on the European market.

Rocco Forte Hotels aren't a household name to South American travellers, but with over 15 European resorts, they've developed a strong brand in the UK & Europe. Compared to the Six Senses brand, now owned by *Intercontinental Hotels Group*, they're recognized more globally than *Rocco Forte Hotels*. However, they still only have 26 locations, being spread across most of the world.

The options to obtain a legacy brand are:
1. License an established brand
2. Acquire 20+ hotels globally, brand them together & refurbish them to the same standard.

A third option is to work with an established brand in another sector. *Bvlgari* is an example of a company that did this. This demonstrates how finding a legacy brand in a transferable industry that speaks to the same group of customers is possible, and it's likely to take a different route to obtain your legacy brand.

The other benefit of a legacy brand is that it already has a massive database of loyal fans and followers that it can tap into. *Bvlgari*, for example, has a vast number of customers who buy luxury products. So bolting a luxury hotel resort onto their product line makes a lot of sense for them, regardless of whether they run it.

ESG

A big driver & influencer of investment now is ESG (Environmental, Society, Governance). In some circles, this is called impact investing. Investors & customers want to know their money is improving the world. Both companies and investors have a directive & a requirement to invest in projects & investments that support the ESG agenda.

Regardless of your thoughts around climate change or similar related narratives, if your customers & investors are willing to direct capital to an ESG-biased product, it makes sense to position your investment requirements in line with this & tap into the funds available. Nobody said you have to sign up for government CBDCs & get a digital tracker in your arm, but creating a business that leaves the planet in a better state is good. It's time someone told the corporate giants to clean up all their waste.

Team

In addition to the day-to-day management of the business, any investor needs to see a high-level management team driving the company when they invest. These are not the people dealing with customers or managing staff. Following is the core leadership team needed:

The Visionary Strategist: This person, typically carrying the CEO title, is responsible for creating the concept & the attraction factor that investors want to be a part of. They are the driver of growth for the business.

The Awareness Maestro: Typically a CMO, the awareness maestro is responsible for raising brand awareness with customers and investors through PR, guerilla marketing, and brand awareness campaigns

The Controller: Typically, the COO is responsible for taking the CEO's big ideas and implementing them while ensuring the business runs smoothly.

The Governor: Typically carrying the CFO title, this is the straight-faced, sensible one. You don't mess around when the Governor is in town. This person is responsible for finance in the business, overseeing all governance areas and ensuring things are always done correctly.

The Guru. Typically carrying the CTO or Technical Director title, the Guru is responsible for keeping on top of the solution, & the latest innovations happening in the industry.

The Advisors: Ideally, you want an experienced team of advisors to support the senior management team. These are people who have already walked the path where you want to go but can also add influence to their network and help the team reach the desired result. The advisors are responsible for questioning the senior management team, to ensure the business continues to be driven in the best interest of the shareholders & broader stakeholders.

The questions to ask for identifying your board of advisors could be:

1. Who has already walked the same path before?
2. Who has a connection to your target customers?
3. Who has a connection to your target investors?
4. Who has experience in the governance of your type of business?

The Big Daddy: The final person to consider is the chairman. This individual is well-rounded in most areas, but their bias is towards growth and strategy. They also typically act as coaches to senior management, particularly the CEO, to help them reach the desired result. Still, their ultimate responsibility is to the shareholders.

Vision

With an inspiring vision of where you want to go, an investor will be inspired to fund your dreams. Nobody is interested in mundane, same-old routines day in and day out. An investor wants to be a part of an inspiring journey that impacts the world. The vision should be rooted in where you are now as a business, but also share a bright opportunity of where you can take the company. It would help if you had a strategy to reach that result when you have the vision. I've noticed that too many businesses expect the investor to provide the vision & strategy, but their job is different.

It's their job to provide the rocket fuel & accelerate you on a journey you're already travelling.

I've shared some ideas in this book, but our model has many pieces at play. Most of these pieces are standalone businesses. For this to work, you'll need a master plan vision of how all the pieces interact and fit together, individual visions and strategies for separate pieces, and a plan for bringing that big vision to life.

The Packaging

What makes an attractive opportunity for an investor? This boils down to five core points.

1. The Why
2. The Exit
3. The Returns
4. The Structure
5. The Risk

The Why: It's sometimes about more than just the money. Most investors want to know they're having an impact on the world. Finding people who share your vision & purpose beyond what you're doing will make it an attractive proposition.

The Exit: Investors need to know they can get their money back in the future. They'll invest much more if they know they can quickly withdraw it. The more liquidity you can provide in the investment vehicle, the more capital you'll be willing to contribute.

The Returns: What makes a good investment return? Perhaps 5% per year? 10% per year? The return has to consider several factors: timescale, risk level, inflation rates, liquidity, and the average rate of return for other investments.

The Structure: The investment vehicle's structure must be as tax-efficient as possible. It is ideally a *'pass-through'* entity with limited liability for investors.

If structuring a charity or non-profit-based vehicle for receiving donations, this should be fully tax deductible for companies, & where possible, provide an *'add back'* facility for donations received from individuals. In the UK, this *'add-back'* facility is called *'Gift Aid'*. The government pays the charity 25% of the total donation value with the Gift Aid facility. This accounts for the income tax the individual pays, as any charity donations are typically made after tax. The entity should also be based in a jurisdiction with solid transparency & governance laws.

The Risk: If you can reduce the level of risk an investor faces, this will improve the attractiveness of the investment. Some ways to do this are to structure part of the capital investment as debt and part as equity. This means that as a debt holder of the business, the investor would receive a proportional share of any assets the business owned in the event of business failure. In this example, if the investor debt contribution makes up 50% of the debt owed to creditors, it would receive 50% of any asset sale proceeds.

A second option is to provide the investor with a lien, charge or mortgage on the asset being invested in, such as a property. Essentially, a lien means they own that asset. One final example of risk reduction might be a staged investment. Rather than the investor providing all capital investment on day one of the project, a *'draw-down'* is done for the investment needed immediately. This can mean the investment period takes 12 months or more before all committed capital is invested.

Asset commercialization

One option for packaging an investable deal is to commercialize a piece of what you already have. We call this Asset commercialization, and in simple terms, it means taking what is currently a stagnant asset on the balance sheet or a cost centre in the business and commercializing it under its own legal entity, to generate new revenue from it. This process transforms it from a cost centre to a profit centre for your business.

I've created an in-depth video on this process, which you can find on my YouTube channel or website. Still, the general process to follow is identifying which assets or overheads you have in the business that might have a commercial demand in the marketplace. These assets or overheads are transferred into a subsidiary business, attracting customers for them and, over time, generating additional profit from them.

Example 1

A company employs a small team of HR professionals to provide recruitment, & training to all its staff. This small team represents a *'non-core'* overhead to the business. The company creates a new subsidiary business, transferring this small team into the new business. The new business, whilst still providing HR support to the company, attracts other customers who need recruitment & training support.

Over time, the new business has grown to three times its original size. It has become an asset for its owners rather than a cost. The profit it generates from the new customers pays for any HR support the owning company needs, meaning the overhead is reduced to zero.

Example 2

An office building with unused space

A company is based in an office space that is too big for its requirements. Reorganizing the building and renting the unused space to other tenants generates additional revenue, reducing property-related costs significantly. I've previously used this strategy, reducing my property expenses to zero.

Example 3

Landowner with unused land

The third example is a landowner who owns 100 acres of unused land. Suppose they don't have the capital to invest in and develop the land for alternative uses. By working in partnership with another company, they create a new subsidiary business to grow food and sell it to the local community. This process earns them a fresh revenue stream from an asset they previously had no use for.

Identify

There isn't a category of perfect investors. Instead, some investors are interested in particular types of investments, sizes, locations, or sectors. When looking for potential funders for your project, each investor will be focused on a specific category and size of investment.

For example, a fictional private equity company's investment criteria state that they invest in *'mid-market technology companies in Western Europe.'* This gives you a clear picture of whether they'd be interested in your type of opportunity.

On many occasions, when you find a suitable investor like this, reaching out to them with the opportunity won't work. Because they get so many pitches sent to them, they typically look for introductions from trusted parties only. This helps filter out 99% of the deals they normally get pitched, as they know the trusted parties will only introduce something that is the type of opportunity they're looking for.

When looking for investors for the hotel project, for example, some investors invest at different stages of the project. The first may invest in the bare land, create a master plan for the site, gain all licenses and approvals, and then sell it to a developer. Other investors only invest during the construction phase of the project. The third type of investor typically invests after the project is complete and the hotel is stabilized, generating revenue.

Depending on the structure, this could be straight after completion & handover, where the property runs on a traditional commercial lease agreement. Alternatively, it might be after the hotel reaches stabilization, which may take 3-5 years after project completion & occupancy rates have reached 70%.

This is usually based on a partnership-style arrangement between the hotel operator & hotel investor. This is because the value of the building is based on the profit generated by it. Maximizing profit from hotel operations as fast as possible is the best strategy.

Ideally, suppose you can find an investor who buys into your vision and reason for doing the project. In that case, this will provide that *'perfect investment partner.'* They may be more flexible in their expectations or how and when the money is invested in the project.

Design

This chapter will examine the most critical factors in planning our community, from identifying the perfect site to reviewing the project's component pieces.

Community masterplan

We need a radical rethink of how we use our properties. We need to rethink how we spend our time.

The COVID lockdowns showed us it was possible to work from home & we don't need to spend an hour sitting in congested traffic daily. Whilst it wasn't perfect, we can take some positives from the experience. I've worked from home since 2011, & I've come to understand what I like about it and things that could be improved. Technology has reached a level where we can achieve most things working remotely, which could be completed in a central workplace.

What would be the best way to operate from a property perspective for our *'island'* concept: a community on an island in the middle of the ocean?

From a high-level perspective, the occupant's lifestyle requirements determine the community's needs. We have to know & understand our customers so we can create what they need.

In my case, I think about creating something that I want because many people share my lifestyle requirements.

Still, it's best to properly analyze who will be using the community when designing it. We'll generally do this by creating a customer avatar.

In a broad sense, we can categorize these needs into five types of property:
1. Early homes
2. Mid-life homes
3. Senior homes
4. Leisure property
5. Workspace property

These five types are designed around the people using them. As we grow older, our needs and way of life change, so staying in a property designed for our needs as 20-year-old students will not suit our lifestyle as 70-year-olds in retirement.

Early Homes: The early homes are for people in their early stages of living away from their parents, through to having their first child. For example, they could be the co-living environment of student housing or the current HMOs (House of Multiple Occupancy). However, suppose we're considering a new community. In that case, I don't believe the HMO product is a great one to incorporate into the plan. You'll agree with me if you've experienced living in this environment.

Most HMOs are designed to maximize profit for the landlord, whilst the occupant is forced to live in a matchbox with LOTS of other people. Some people have compared this type of living environment to a squat. This model is a perfect breeding ground to create angry, frustrated people - similar to caged lions.

By grouping like-minded people, they can access people with the same interests, build connections, and work together.

The early homes act as a transitional space, from leaving their parents' house to starting their mid-life home.

Mid-life Homes: Mid-life homes are for people in their mid-stages of life, with or without families. They offer more living space and connections to others in their social circle. By grouping people in the same areas, there's less need for travel to socialize.

Senior Homes: Senior homes are for people in the retirement age group. The current solution for retirement-age housing is not great. It's either retirement villages, in the form of a block of apartments containing people of the same age group, or another option, sheltered housing & nursing homes. My parents are in their mid-60s, so they fit the perfect age bracket for the retirement villages, but that's the last place they'd want to go at this stage. The current solutions are more like a conveyor belt, where people go whilst they wait to die.

Since I was a child, the notion was that you work your whole life & then when you retire, you do all sorts of exciting things, like going on world cruises, & exploring places. To think my parents would go & isolate themselves in a small one-bedroom apartment is far from the truth. Your brain age is the average of the people you surround yourself with. You can stick around a bunch of 80-year-olds doing jigsaw puzzles & waiting to die, or you can be around your grandkids. Which option will make you live longest & be happier?

When people retire, they need to keep their minds active. By cooping yourself up in a retirement flat, it's impossible to keep your mind active by looking at four walls all day, watching TV & doing jigsaw puzzles. Older people don't need a five-bedroom house like they needed 30 years earlier. But they need a home on a single floor, within easy walking distance from their family and social circle. This needs to be a low-maintenance home, all on one level, but something that resembles an element of leisure.

These peoples' roles in the wider community are as *mentors* and guides to the other age groups. A two-bedroom house with a garage & a garden area, with access to care in their home should they need it.

Multi-generational homes are something people will move toward over the next two decades. This is how other cultures live, but Western society has moved away from it over the past century, increasingly preferring to isolate themselves. This may encompass everything from the three types we've discussed, packaging them into a large enough home to accommodate three or more generations of a family.

Rather than being a standalone house where everyone from the extended family lives, it might be three or four properties within a larger plot. This option might work better for those who don't like spending time in close quarters with their interfering mother-in-law.

This same result can still be achieved within a private village without squeezing everyone into the same plot of land. The private village is designed to include all three groups within a few minute's walking distance. This model enables everyone in the family to maintain their level of privacy.

Leisure Property: Leisure property is essential when considering the *'island community'* model. Firstly, it brings external revenue into the community from outsiders, such as through a hotel, spa, or sporting facilities. Secondly, it creates a space for entertainment & a reason for the community to gather, whether at a restaurant, a cafe, on the golf course, or just a central meeting place like a village square, gardens, a park, or a music venue.

Sports Facilities: Besides those meeting places, we also have needs to satisfy. We need to fill our time with activities. This could include a tennis club, a golf course, a child play area, football & rugby pitches, basketball courts, and a theatre event space.

Then we need to think about other fitness needs. Everyone in the community needs a way to stay active & fit. This can be achieved with a gym, including outdoor walking paths, cycle paths & running tracks. If the landscape accommodates it, it could be something more unique, like a climbing wall.

Workspace: Next, we must think about how we work every day. The current model of commuting to a company office or working from home full time is not the answer to a workplace problem. Having a co-working style hub within the community is probably the hybrid compromise between the two extremes in which Western countries currently find themselves.

This hybrid workspace needs to be within easy walking distance of the housing & adjacent to the central community space, which encourages people flow & activity in that central public area. Within the workspace facility, this could include the shared desk concept of a traditional co-working space and more private office space for those who want it. It could also have meeting & conference space and facilities for others to visit from outside the community, thus creating additional revenue streams for the project.

Within our longer-term model of investing in local businesses, this workspace could also be an incubator space for those we've invested in. This creates more jobs for the indigenous locals, too.

If we combine this workspace concept with education space, changing our education model would dramatically change how we use the space, & how much space is needed. But if the nursery or school were next door to our office too, would that make more sense, especially considering the more blended view of learning we'll talk about in the other chapters of the book? Ultimately, suppose the working week changed to four-day weeks and the fifth day was used for continued learning & education.

In that case, the traditional workspace could be re-utilized as the education space, meaning we wouldn't need extra buildings dedicated solely to education. The central concept around the workspace property is to remove that daily commute time whilst being a better alternative to working from home.

Community Hub: A sustainable community space must include all facets of a functioning community. Many private community concepts only focus on a particular design or style of a housing unit, forgetting about everything that makes a community function. This is partly intentional due to the extra cost of creating this supporting infrastructure.

Second, unless you're experienced in designing cities, it's just something that you don't think about until you wake up in your new community, & you don't have anywhere to go.
The third reason they're omitted is that people rely on the government to provide this.

In addition to housing units that suit different age groups, communal spaces for meeting friends are also required. Community hubs are also important, whether a village hall or central event space. In the UK village economy, pubs have served this purpose for centuries because they've acted as that central meeting place for community members.

Medical Facilities: Whilst you may be able to use the medical facilities close to your community, if these aren't available or you've created your community on an actual physical island, you'll need emergency medical support.

You can collaborate with other communities or *'islands'*, sharing a central facility. It may only be a small building used for treating the most critical issues, such as snake bites or emergency first aid. This topic needs serious consideration in how you'll manage any medical situation.

Food Garden: If we're growing our food garden within the community, this additional space requirement will need to be factored in, as well as both a growth area and a storage and prep area. This can serve a dual purpose: as a place for community members to meet or relax in nature.

Masterplan Layout: While many people have heard of using feng shui in their buildings to create better *'flow'*, few have heard about sacred geometry and its benefits. Rather than using sacred geometry on a single building, though, we use it to design the entire community layout. Multiple studies and research have shown that this is healthy for all its occupants and can increase food growth yields, where a community grows its own food.

Capacity Planning: Looking at the whole project as a 100-year development plan, each with its phases of development, we need to design in extra capacity for growth & expansion. Whilst many communities are designed with today's requirements in mind, if the design is successful & truly sustainable, people will stay long-term & grow their families there. This could lead to the community accommodating three or four generations of the same family.

With four generations living in the community, this means an 8x growth if each generation had two children. So, the ability to grow the community by 8x is a critical design factor in making a genuinely sustainable & long-term choice.

Site selection

Next, we have to consider location. If you already have a site, some factors will be out of your control. The factors we'll discuss are those we consider when selecting a hotel location. However, the same rules also provide a good baseline for community development. These are not listed in order of preference.

Taxation: How attractive is the location for taxation purposes? What incentives are there to attract investment into the area? Are there any special economic zones that could be used? Let's look at other places globally, like the UAE.

From implementing strong investment incentives, millions of investors have set up residences & invested there in the last thirty years.

As well as investment-related taxation, we also consider any taxes that might be appropriate after the investment. Is the location favourable for operating a business there? What taxes are being imposed on a company? Import tax? Export tax? Sales tax? Employer taxes? Corporation tax? Capital gains tax? All these dictate the location's attractiveness for setting up a community or business there. What about personal taxes? If we invest in local businesses, this might affect our tax rates, too. If individual tax rates are high, this limits how attractive the opportunity is, & therefore, how much money will be invested.

Residency: The next thing to consider is citizenship & residency options. Suppose we're building a hotel, investing in a business, or creating a community.

In that case, we ideally want the option of obtaining citizenship, or at the very least, long-term residency, with the option of gaining citizenship later. Caribbean islands receive so much investment because of their citizenship & residency programs. Combine these with low taxation, & you've created the perfect baseline for attracting overseas capital.

Political Stability: The following criterion we look for is political stability. Is the country stable, or is it going through a civil war? I've been offered many opportunities in paradise locations. Still, the government has very low political stability in these cases. I hope these countries sort themselves out, & the opportunity to invest will appear.

Low Crime: One of the rising issues is whether it's safe to visit a particular location. In the UK, crime is on the rise. Gangs are taking over the streets in some cities, scammers are constantly one step ahead, & paedophiles are infiltrating our education system.

That's why finding a location with a low crime level is so important. Various platforms publish data on crime levels in each area; one platform is Numbeo, who publish the crime & safety index, enabling you to search by town, city, or country. This divides different crime types into individual categories, with each category ranking separately.

For example, murder statistics are ranked differently to corruption. It shares actual data rather than just presenting it similarly to a leaderboard ranking system. This lets you see how safe locals perceive the area to be. This data reports how many crimes per 1,000 inhabitants in the area.

Most people say certain countries are dangerous without visiting them or viewing the data. For example, all countries in Africa are perceived as being very dangerous based solely on Western media stories.

However, there are countries in Africa that you've probably never heard of, which are some of the safest in the world.

One of the downsides of developing countries is the high level of corruption. The corruption score should also be low, but while not ideal, this would rule out many otherwise perfect countries from the list. I'm still determining the reason behind corruption, but I heard about someone stopped by the police in Ghana for speeding. The police officer concerned suggested that the driver pay him the equivalent of USD $7 and that he'd forget all about the incident. To the policeman, this amount would likely feed his family for a few days, but to the Western tourist, it was just pocket change. This wouldn't happen as frequently if locals were given decent opportunities, and they wouldn't feel like turning to crime.

High customer demand: Any business you will create or invest in at the new community location needs access to high customer demand.

If you're exporting products, the company needs access to these customers. For example, if you're exporting coffee beans, you'll need easy access to transport the beans. If you don't have the logistics and infrastructure, it'll be challenging from day one. Likewise, if we're looking at sites for a hotel resort, a location with high tourism demand for our product offering is vital. It also needs supporting infrastructure, including other tourist attractions and activities. Whilst you can't guarantee making a sale, you can verify that people want to buy your type of offering in that location.

Additionally, verifying demand for your specific offering is essential. For example, when we look at locations for a resort, we want to find somewhere that already has at least one five-star resort, ideally one of the legacy brands. You can be a frontier seeker & create the first business of its type in the new location, but this presents a much greater risk.

To be successful, a frontier seeker may have to do much of the industry or country promotion yourself that otherwise would have been done by your forerunners. Creating customer demand from zero might involve investing millions of dollars into TV advertising & marketing campaigns. This is what governments & legacy brands do. This additional process means a much more extended period for the business to reach the stabilization stage, where it can generate sufficient income to pay its running costs.

Access to resources: As well as physical products & construction materials, another valuable resource we need is people with the right skill sets & experience. We might have big ambitions to create an architectural masterpiece. Still, if we need more skills to build it locally, we'll need to bring those skills from elsewhere.

Where will we find the labour force if it's not from local people?

Likewise, if we build the project on an island in the middle of the ocean, how might we get those resources to the island? Whenever you have to bring in external resources, whether people or products, it adds enormous complexity & costs to the project and other logistical nightmares like arranging visas, etc.

In the past, our company was involved in building a school on a remote island off the west coast of Scotland. The project was only a few miles from the mainland but didn't have vehicle ferries to reach it. This meant transporting everything and everyone on a small fishing boat, then physically handling it from the boat onto the pier, and then carrying all construction equipment, materials & tools by hand for about half a mile to the site location. Compared to doing the same project on the mainland, the costs & time it took were about eight times larger.

The same principles apply to a hotel project. After construction, the hotel must be run by experienced people, such as chefs, & management staff. While local people can be trained in these roles, this takes time, so in the interim, they must be filled from an external labour pool if those skill sets aren't already present in the community. In that example, we must also consider the logistics involved in bringing these resources in from externally. Where will a team of chefs live? Will we need to build separate accommodation for these people or resources?

Lastly, is a training program available in the area, such as a technical college, to help you train new staff?

If not, we may need to set up our own training school, creating it as part of the broader support ecosystem.

Import taxes: We've talked about this already, but an essential factor in choosing a location is how much it might cost to import materials.

Whilst our model is to buy as much as possible from local people, specific items or equipment will likely be unavailable from the local people. For example, furniture, commercial kitchen equipment, and vehicles must be imported from another country. How much tax will be paid on these items when we import them? Finding a location with low import taxes is a significant factor.

Suitable Infrastructure: Whilst it seems obvious, we need the essential infrastructure for a hotel business. Travelling 100 miles from a country's airport might take days or weeks without roads. A gravel road is the minimum standard, but these tend to get washed away or become impassable during the rainy season. A sealed surface road is an excellent standard to look for.

The next vital piece of infrastructure is an international airport. Does the location have an airport that can be reached quickly, or is it only reachable by boat?

Whether we're building projects or running a hotel, if it takes three days to reach the nearest transport hub, this will significantly reduce the project's chance of success.

Finally, we need to think about direct flights. Where are the target customers/investors travelling from? If people buy one of the houses in our new community, where are they based already, and which countries might they wish to travel to for day-to-day and work-life commitments? Having direct flights from these locations is very important.

I can only speak about my preferences, but I'm not too fond of the travel process when going anywhere. It is such a waste of my time; it's tedious & inconvenient. If I'm travelling somewhere, I want to get there as fast as possible, hassle-free, & convenient as possible. I hate waiting around; I hate needing to transfer between different forms of transport.

The ideal scenario for me is to fly point to point, & be where I need to be, ideally taking no more than 8 hours in total travel time. The need to wait around in travel lounges whilst I wait for a connecting flight or other transport is just frustrating. Having a direct flight is the minimum criterion for our projects.

Making it easy for people to get there with as few connections as possible is essential. I've looked at travelling to some countries from the UK; travelling to Africa, one country, might take 8 hours flying direct, whereas a neighbouring country with no direct flight can take 30 hours, connecting through various other countries along the way.

Lastly, being less than 90 minutes from the international airport to your location is also essential when you're in a country. Suppose there's nothing suitable within that travel radius. Pushing it to a two-hour travel radius is doable in that case.

However, this probably has to be the limit and should also be weighed against the total time spent travelling from the departure countries.

Low bureaucracy red tape: Western economies are considered favourable toward doing business, but this is becoming less common. Over the last decade, we've seen more red tape & bureaucracy creeping in, with new legislation making it complex and more costly for small businesses to operate.

This is an example from which other less developed countries can benefit. Specific industries need regulations to protect the people, and good food hygiene and health and safety practices should be followed to protect everyone. However, regulations and legislation mustn't go too far, created to generate even more work and cost to business. Suppose we use other locations outside Western economies as a suitable benchmark.

In that case, places like Singapore and the UAE offer a low *'red tape'* environment in which to operate your business. Of course, there might be a direct correlation between high taxes & lots of red tape.

Strong legal system: Any chosen location should have a robust and transparent legal system. For example, when buying a property in a foreign country, we must ensure nobody can steal or confiscate it.

Industry support: When we invest in or create a business, we want to know that there's a support ecosystem to help us; we don't want to make everything we need from zero. All industries have specific regulations & guidance to follow, for example, & we want to know we've got those practices correct in that location. If we're constructing a property, we'll need to comply with local building regulations & laws. If a country doesn't have these basic guidelines, it's in the too early stage and presents a high risk of failure.

I saw an example of this on a Caribbean island. Someone had built themselves a considerable-sized mansion about ten years previous. A few years later, someone purchased the plot next door & built a large industrial factory. In the developed world, this doesn't happen because zoning laws prevent people from building whatever they want in specific locations. This is a fundamental level of regulation that needs to be in place, which you'd consider a supporting function. You wouldn't want to build a five-star hotel and then find someone next door to start mining for coal.

Another example of industry support is having industry associations for each type of business in your location. For instance, I'd like to see an association set up to help hospitality businesses. Still, I also want to see a government department created to support the industry by promoting it through various marketing campaigns. We see this in countries like Rwanda, where their *'Visit Rwanda'* campaign actively promotes the country as a destination.

Attitude toward opportunity: The next one is something you'll never find statistics on. Different cultures have varying attitudes toward opportunities. In the Western economies, for example, people find excuses not to do things. In contrast, in more developing countries, my experience of these places shows people generally have a *'we can do anything'* attitude. The UK's attitude toward opportunity has been negative for a long time.

About 25 years ago, I worked with someone who, when I presented him with an opportunity to work on a project together, rejected the idea with, *'Who do you think you are? You're not Richard Branson'*. This attitude sums up the British public now; only a small percentage of people are willing to 'rise above their station'. So, finding a location with the right attitude toward opportunity is essential. It'll also determine whether you can find suitable, motivated staff & a supply chain to help you.

A country where its population lives on some guaranteed income, such as universal basic income, would reduce the drive to achieve anything in life.

Low competition: We've discussed having proven demand for our businesses' product offerings, but we also need to consider how much competition there is already. High competition means struggling to get customers, with potentially low-profit margins. An example of this is Mauritius.

The majority of hotel resortsin Mauritius are five-star resorts. Just about every legacy five-star brand has a presence there. This represents high competition because you're fighting with established locations to be seen by new customers. Now, you can create something very niche within your product offering, making it a destination location less reliant on the general tourist trade, but that's a subject for another book.

The ideal location choice should have that proven demand as Mauritius does, but it'll have low competition. It's a delicate balance between the two. The bi-product is an ecosystem of staff & supporting businesses that are already in place because they're already supporting those existing businesses.

Investment ecosystem: Ideally, there'll be a supportive investment ecosystem in place, for example, a stock exchange with transparency & audit requirements. This provides a vehicle for creating a publicly traded vehicle, which makes it easier to attract external investment. It gives transparency & the ability to invest in companies, whether in an earlier stage or later, as a public company listing. Earlier-stage ecosystems like Mauritius have created their stock exchange, and again, we can see why they're one of the most attractive markets in the African region to invest in.

No export or sales tax: To attract revenue for our model, the businesses we create or invest in rely on revenue outside that local ecosystem. This means that export taxes have to be low, ideally zero. Also, sales taxes have to be low or zero. One of the biggest problems for industries such as hospitality is the businesses aren't just competing against local competitors; they're also competing against companies in other countries, all based solely on how much sales tax or *'tourist tax'* is added to a customer's bill in each jurisdiction.

Suppose one country is 10% cheaper, based on having lower sales tax. In that case, it'll attract revenue from these customers who otherwise might have travelled to that more expensive country. A government must play the long game to attract outside investment. The long game for a government tax department is to encourage investment, encourage spending, create jobs, create money circulation, and stop trying to strangle the goose before it's laid the egg.

If money circulates in the economy, people buy things from within that economy. But strangle the economy, & none of that money circulation happens. Instead, cash flows to places that can think at a higher level of consciousness.

Government Assistance: Whilst I'm generally not a fan of governments, I'm always open to working with a government that has the foresight to see the bigger picture & work on behalf of the people's best interest. With everything in this current state of being, we'll need some level of government interaction to achieve our objectives. This means we're inclined to look for a location where the local government is motivated to help us achieve what we want.

For example, I recently contacted several government officials in various African nations, looking for assistance from them to help us locate local businesses within their country. Out of the six countries I contacted, only two replied.

The first representative told me I must engage a consultant to compile a list of suitable businesses. In contrast, the second representative sent me a list of local businesses at no charge. We can see from this example which is the most likely to offer us the assistance we need to achieve our goals should we invest in those countries.

Natural Resources & Environment: It's essential, when considering a location or site, to understand what natural resources and advantages it has, either on that site or from the wider local community. For example, what is the climate like? Is it an arid desert, is it a tropical rainforest, or is it in a cold, snowy climate? How many hours of sunlight does the site receive each day? Does it have a flowing clean water source, such as a stream or a waterfall, that you can tap into?

What are wind levels like? Is it suitable for using wind to power your community? Is the wind too strong?

Would it pose a threat to your buildings and infrastructure? What weather events occur in the location? For example, is it in the hurricane belt, does it suffer from cyclones, is there a tsunami risk, or is there an active volcano nearby? Does it get affected by earthquakes? Does it have a supply of seawater?

Is there timber on the site? What food sources does the site have? What type of soil is present? It may be all sand. Will growing anything in the ground be possible, or will you need to consider something else?

Ground Types: What is the ground consistency? Is it sand, is it soil, is it clay, is it peat, or is it marshland? Or perhaps it's rock. Each ground type will offer advantages and disadvantages, depending on your plans. While rock provides a solid base to build on, if you need to level it or dig below surface level, this will be a long, costly job of chiselling the rock out.

Likewise, I was offered a site in a paradise location next to the beach. The problem was that the ground was all sand. Whilst it's not impossible to build on sand, as they have in other locations like Dubai, this is a lot more expensive to build on.

One last point is who owns the mineral rights for the land. The last thing we want to happen is to build a private village, and then someone comes along & starts digging for oil because they own the rights to the land. Who has rights over the surrounding sea area if the site is next to the beach? Can someone erect an oil drilling platform right in front of your resort?

Tourism Support: If planning to build a hotel or spa resort, will the location support this type of business? For example, are local attractions giving guests something to do? What is the scenery like? Is it next to a beach or in the middle of an urban city?

Size Requirements: Next, we must consider the site's required size. Is it big enough for what we need? As a guide from our perspective, if we're considering a hotel resort, our target is to build a resort with up to 100 keys. Room sizes are generally 60-150 sq meters each, with public areas around the same size as the total room floor area, as a basic rule of thumb. If building a spa, this has a minimum floor area of 1,000 square meters. Then, we have to consider outside space.

For a private village, we generally look at the village to contain about 100 houses, & 100 apartments. In addition to the residence floor area, we must include space for facilities and the central village area. The density must be low with all of our developments. For example, I don't want to live in a house where properties overlook each other in the development. This means allowing at least one acre of ground for each home. If we build a golf course, it generally needs about 200-300 acres for the standard course, & other facilities we want to create.

Additionally, we need a site large enough to house the supporting functions; for example, we need to consider the *'back office'* roles of a village or hotel resort, like the laundry and maintenance workshop. We also need enough space to grow food, generate electricity, and deal with waste treatment. As a general guide, we're looking for a site with at least 1,000 acres for a private village, including a resort.

If we convert an existing site, it must be large enough to expand. For example, suppose we find an existing hotel resort that we can upgrade. In that case, the hotel must have enough land capacity to expand to 100 keys and house all the previously mentioned facilities without feeling overdeveloped.

Suppose a government aligns with the criteria set out in this chapter. In that case, its people will be much happier with the country's leaders. Investors have these requirements, so a government can either accommodate them or continue with the same problems it's had for centuries.

Optimized

This chapter will examine the project's infrastructure components, including the buildings, energy generation, water sources, and waste disposal, from a sustainability perspective.

Property

Shelter is one of humankind's foundational needs. That shelter may be a canvas tent or a mountain log cabin. Achieving that foundational need has two problems.

First, the average person can't afford a property unless they take on debt. Debt shackles the individual to a lifetime of slavery. The second problem is the product, which we'll look at now.

When we talk about *'the product'*, we mean the actual property. Have you noticed how poorly constructed new homes are these days? Paper-thin walls divide up rooms you can barely fit furniture into, never mind living in. The gardens are tiny, surrounded by a 2-meter flimsy wood panel fence, overlooked by every house in the street.

In the UK, we have housing estates where properties are so tightly packed together that it's barely legal to call them *'detached'*. The average Victorian house has rooms larger than the entire floor area of these newly built houses.

I must be the only person on the planet who has an issue with how ugly buildings have become in the last 50 years—ugly square boxes with no character. In search of architects for my project, I looked disappointingly at about 800 practices and their past projects. Whatever happened to architecture, being about creating beautiful buildings? A three-year-old toddler could design a building with more character than most of the firms I've looked at. Has the architecture industry lost its passion for the job?

Many people won't like me saying this, but 95% of the architects I looked at had bog-standard designs—basic square boxes—bland, characterless, and ugly, with zero imagination. Why not create something you can be proud of putting your name to? We don't want boring boxes; we want characterful buildings by which we can feel inspired.

Drive through most historic towns in the UK, & you'll see a whole lot of horrible ugly buildings along most high streets.

In historic market towns, where you'd expect to see ancient buildings, these have been left to decay whilst being surrounded by buildings constructed in the 70s, 80s & 90s, all in a state of disrepair, with very little maintenance ever performed on them.

There are some exceptions. There's a small minority of towns and villages where the planners have forced developers to build well-designed buildings in keeping with the existing property heritage. However, these tend to be in the most expensive locations because I suppose they must believe the rest of the country is just where the peasants live.

Methods & materials

In our island community, we don't have spare resources to waste on maintaining & rebuilding, duplicating our efforts over & over again.

Rather than just considering the upfront cost of initial construction, we must consider the entire lifecycle cost of our choice of materials. That means, rather than installing something with a 12-month warranty because, it's the cheapest option. Instead, we install something with a 30-year guarantee that might cost 10% more but does not need ongoing maintenance.

Using a life cycle costing method, we measure the upfront cost, ongoing maintenance costs & replacement costs over a fixed period of, say, 100 years, as well as any additional or knock-on costs it might have, such as increased energy usage. When considering the lifecycle cost for every option, we consider what effects our choice might have on other elements of the build or our master plan in general.

It's funny: I watched a *Grand Designs* episode on TV a few months ago. In this episode, someone built a house for himself that was *'energy neutral'*.

By that, he'd designed it so it didn't need heating or cooling, and its power source came from a solar panel, so it cost him ZERO to run his building. If it can be done for one house, that model can be scaled up to suit all buildings in a community. It all comes down to designing the buildings with the right intention.

The cost of constructing buildings will reduce significantly as robotics enter the industry. The transition to robotics won't happen immediately; it will first move to an entirely offsite/modular build model, delivered through a production line, similar to how cars are built. As I write this, in 2024, the modular production route is being adopted massively across new build construction.

As this model is perfected, we'll slowly see the introduction of robotics, just like we saw with car manufacturing in the 1990s. In Western economies, the labour element of the build process makes up a significant portion of the total build cost.

When robotics entirely takes over the process, it'll reduce the build cost by 80%, with a house being constructed in days rather than months if constructed the traditional way.

Will this lead to job loss in the construction industry? No, probably not, because the construction industry has suffered colossal staff shortages for at least 30 years. During every recession, more people leave the industry for better-paying jobs, & currently, we're seeing the baby boomer generation all leaving the industry by 2030.

Whilst I'm not a fan of the modular construction industry, it offers construction workers a very low quality of work experience & variety, essentially being a temporary workforce until robotics are powerful enough to take over completely.

If I were advising the construction industry, I'd recommend either moving into modular offsite manufacturing or specializing in one of the niches of construction where robotics can't go right now, such as restoring historic buildings.

Eventually, robotics will replace every manual role. However, focusing on building conservation is a bit like the specialist car services industry, where you have very niche specialist garages that restore classic cars or do specialist performance tuning. They make significantly more money than a standard garage that might provide more general services like vehicle inspections and repairs.

The next evolution of the construction process is a shift to 3d printing. This means setting up a jig at the construction site, where a 3d printer will *print* the building. If successful, we'll see this model being used more readily by 2030. This removes the remaining elements of the cost involved in transportation & materials.

If such a technology can be used on such a large scale, this could make the construction industry, as we currently know it, redundant. Ultimately, the building would be free after paying for the 3d printing equipment, its source materials (the printer *'ink'*) and the land. As it's *'printed'* on-site, there are no transportation costs either, and with this model, it can construct a house in less than three days.

Our living space

Did you know that research says our environment dictates our mindset, and our mindset dictates how the brain works and how we perceive our world?

Do you think it's just a coincidence that those inner-city communities, the tightly packed council estates, the areas with no gardens, are also those with the lowest paid workers, the highest crime rates, and the highest levels of mental health issues?

Take the garden analogy. If you don't have a nice

view or a nice *'outlook'* from your kitchen window,

perhaps you won't have a *'nice outlook'* toward

your life aspirations. The system is designed to

suppress a large portion of the population, thinking

small and worrying about their hamster wheel

existence.

I've lived in this environment twice during my adult

life: in two separate cities in the UK. Both times, my

mental state dropped; it was a very dense energy

as if something was pushing me down. It's a bizarre

sensation to describe. Thinking long-term or with a

sense of vision or clarity was challenging, and my

thoughts were clouded.

You wouldn't be reading this book if I still lived in

either of those houses now. Likewise, if I can see

for miles when I'm somewhere with open scenery,

my ideas flow continuously.

So, any property solution must include good-sized living areas, good-sized gardens, and lots of privacy. Following the feng shui methodology, any workspace should also be divided between the five areas of flow to let people work at their optimum level of performance.

Ongoing disrepair

The third issue with the current property stock and building method is that they're designed to guarantee future work for the construction and property maintenance industry.

Through constant maintenance and ongoing replacement, building lifecycle costs are enormous and prevent us from reaching that *property freedom'* we aspire to. Let me give you an example.

During my career, I've been involved in various property development projects, from building new homes, renovating hotels, building offices, building schools, or renovating ancient manor houses & castles. I've noticed something very different between these old buildings and those built more recently. The historic buildings need much less maintenance over their lifespan. One example is the windows. Many of these buildings have the original window frames fitted since the day it was constructed 300 years ago.

Compared to more modern buildings, despite regular maintenance, the windows are rotten and need replacement in less than 30 years. My parents built a house in 1995, and despite regular maintenance on those window frames, 20 years later, at least two of those frames were rotten. You could have opted for PVC windows, but will PVC last 300 years? What do we do with all that waste plastic when it comes time to replace it anyway?

This constant need to maintain our buildings, whether residential, commercial, industrial, or agricultural, is like taking two steps forward and one step back, always being dragged back from making progress when we should be able to build it and then forget about it.

I sometimes feel that the materials we're forced to use are designed to create that ongoing maintenance workload. This keeps the economic machine growing, which raises prices and drives the need for borrowing even more debt.

In 2018, a technology company approached me, seeking investment to develop further a new product they'd been working on. They'd created a product that didn't need maintenance over its lifespan. This product was a commercial fire system. For context, a commercial fire system is typically installed in commercial buildings such as hotels, offices, care homes, etc, and it's used to detect fire in the buildings.

These systems generally need to be maintained and regularly tested, with the individual parts lasting less than ten years.

This has created its specialist industry, one that we were previously a part of, with our contracting business, so I understand this product completely.

When the business approached me, I was still in the headspace of believing the traditional way of doing things was the best, and should this product be rolled out to the mainstream, it would wipe out an entire industry, leaving thousands of engineers unemployed. I believed the product would be bad for the human race.

Six years later, I think removing that need for regular maintenance reduces the cost to those businesses where it's used. Rather than paying for maintenance, a company can invest those savings into other business areas.

This removes the cost burden from our daily life. Much of our systems are designed to create an ongoing cost or reliance, as this is the only way the existing systems can survive. They need to keep feeding themselves.

Eliminating those ongoing financial commitments allows us to live at a much lower cost. Unnecessary costs are just more shackles keeping us chained to the system. If our hotel doesn't have to replace parts, the business generates more profit, which can be reinvested in other projects. Most importantly, we aren't sending our money to a faraway land, benefitting some faceless corporate entity. The money stays local.

Considering the potential unemployment impact this practice would have, it will take a long time for the *new* practices to be implemented. Most people don't like change, especially when there's a significant cost of replacement that comes with that change.

In this example of the fire system, it takes 15-20 years to be fully implemented in most commercial buildings. Let's consider the high level of retirement & people reskilling into other careers versus the very low number of new career entrants. There probably isn't an unemployment issue.

There wouldn't be a cost if we didn't need to maintain our buildings. We can invest that money more proactively to improve our lives.

Smart buildings

Are smart buildings good for humanity and our freedom mission? While the controllers will sell you a glorious picture of how smart buildings and smart cities are part of a utopian society, I will tell you the truth. Anyone who says Smart cities are great doesn't understand the technology or why it's being implemented. Smart cities are not for your benefit as a citizen. They're focused on surveillance and control.

While they're presented as a solution to better traffic flow, & reduced carbon emissions, we don't need self-driving cars to be free.

We need fewer people trying to control us, telling us how we should live, act or be. The theory of a smart building can be good, but it can also be just as terrifying as its larger smart city uncle. Imagine a fridge that reorders your food automatically, so you don't have to visit the supermarket. Sounds good, but what if that fridge was the only access to food you had, & one day, it just stopped reordering it for you? Does it sound like a fantasy? This technology already exists, but a smart grid needs to be developed to function.

The smart grid & those who control it can dictate whether that device can function when you need it to. The same applies to your TV or smart devices, smartphone, and even your access to the internet.

If you've been a naughty boy in the eyes of the government, switching off your device from the outside world is very easy. That can also mean switching off your bank account. Ultimately, the government dictators, along with their corporate paymasters, want complete control over their slave population. You don't feel like working today? Call in sick? Don't worry; they'll have an app connected to your skin to tell them if you're lying. Bad luck, you'd better get your ass to work unless you want to lose some privileges.

There are benefits to smart buildings, though. Still, they existed long before anyone talked about smart cities or IOT (Internet of Things).

So, where do we draw the line between what's good and what's bad? The easiest way is to say that any control system, device, or sensor connected to the outside world isn't good and should be avoided. Anything internal should be okay.

Let's consider a few beneficial examples. How about the sensors that turn your lights off when nobody's around? They save your electricity and cannot be controlled externally (unless it's connected to Wi-Fi). If you can control it from your phone, so can they!!!

How about a vacuum system that sucks crumbs off the carpet by using a sensor in your skirting boards to sense when foreign objects have fallen on the carpet. This means you never have to vacuum again. This would be a good thing; it frees up your time from doing these mundane maintenance tasks, and there's no reason for it to be connected to the outside world.

Regarding smart home systems, it's best to avoid a Wi-Fi network and anything that connects to Wi-Fi. If you need an internet connection to work or stream TV, it's best to use a hard-wired line that you can unplug.

Wi-Fi is bad for our health because it emits an electromagnetic field. This means that anything emitting an EMF should also be placed on that *'naughty list'*, & be treated with caution or avoided altogether. As many people already know, our mobile phones are equally bad for us. Still, we continue to carry them around all day in our pockets, literally frying our reproductive organs. The wireless earphones people have adopted are equally bad for damaging our health. If people continue to use these devices, we'll see a massive increase in brain tumour cases. If we want to go even deeper, even the power cables around our homes emit an EMF.

The building fabric

The next thing we need to look at is the building fabric. What is the building constructed of, & what's the construction method? A modern method of construction used in Western countries is passive house construction. Theoretically, the house has to be airtight so heat can't escape.

The problem with this method is that the building becomes so airtight that nothing can get in, and nothing can get out. Now, as soon as you add moisture to the internal space, whether through breathing, wet clothing, wet towels, taking a shower, etc, suddenly you've got moisture inside the building that can't escape, which subsequently creates mould.

Now, the happy clappers of this building method will say that so long as a good ventilation system is present and working, mould won't cause problems.

The problem with this assumption and my argument is that it relies on the ventilation system always working perfectly for the rest of the building's life. When one component breaks in that ventilation system, moisture sticks and cannot escape. How often do you notice whether your bathroom fan works to its full design capacity?

Better alternative building methods are available that let the building fabric breathe naturally. This means moisture can leave the building without causing dampness or mould issues. Hemp construction is just one method, but there are many more natural ways to build. In addition to being healthier for the building's occupants, they're also more sustainable and don't damage the environment either.

Industrial hemp has many uses. In addition to constructing buildings, it can be used to make insulation, soap, clothing, bioplastics, and food sources. Over 25,000 different products are made using hemp.

The energy framework

The problem with the current energy supply system is that it's been developed to make a small group of people extremely wealthy.

Entire industries have been funded, developed & entrenched themselves in our day-to-day lives. When alternative models or energy sources have been discovered, these have been suppressed, stolen, or just put out of business.

In the late 1800s, Nikola Tesla invented a device to create free electricity. As with all inventions, they needed funding to roll them out to the world. So Nikola Tesla teamed up with Thomas Edison in a quest to gain funding & roll out his invention to the world. Unfortunately, Thomas Edison wasn't batting for the same team, & already in the pockets of J.P Morgan, & John Rockefeller, they stole the patents from Nikola Tesla's inventions, then suppressed them, not to be seen until recently. This happened because JP Morgan & John Rockefeller were the primary owners of the oil industry & they didn't want anyone to come in & take away their kingdom by providing free energy devices.

The same has happened countless times with other inventions and businesses that have *'been buried'*. Of course, they've recently used much more covert tactics by introducing legislation that removes potential upstarts and disruptors from the market, limiting who can compete.

Even the current patent system is designed this way: Endless paperwork, expensive lawyers, red tape, bureaucracy, lengthy submission and approval processes, and legislative hoops to jump through. This carries a substantial upfront cost, so any *'small inventor'* can't afford to obtain patents. Sometimes, people from those competing industries also approve or decline the patent approval process.

Then we have subsidies in the market, provided by governments & NGOs, making it even harder for *'an alternative'* to compete. Take the example of *Tesla* cars. As a company, *Tesla* has never made a profit from selling its vehicles. Yet, it's one of the most valuable companies on the planet.

The only reason it's survived this long is due to the subsidies & government contracts it's received. It only gets these subsidies because the *WEF* and similar organizations push their climate change agenda.

Electric vehicles have existed for over a century. Photographic evidence shows cars being powered by electricity in the late 1800s. Again, these were suppressed by groups who controlled the oil interests. So, technology has remained low-key, though we can see it easily just by looking at a golf cart or milk floats from the 1960s and 1970s. I'm not an advocate for electric vehicles, but I use this example to demonstrate how solutions get suppressed unless it suits someone's agenda to promote them, normally as another tool for control.

Suppose new, better technologies were put on an equal playing field without all the *'agenda pleasing'* subsidies.

In that case, we'd see a very different picture.
Currently, suppose your solution benefits someone
else's agenda. In that case, you'll receive countless
subsidies and support. Still, if it doesn't serve those
interests, your competitor will receive that support
instead.

If you look at how energy is delivered currently,
let's take gas as an example. It's taken from the
ground and piped to an energy processing plant.
The gas is ignited and burnt, which generates
electricity. The electricity is distributed through
cables and into our buildings. I've oversimplified it a
lot, but you get the point.

The costs involved in that process are:

1. Finding the gas source (exploration)
2. Piping the gas
3. Equipment to convert from gas to electricity
4. Cabling to distribute electricity
5. Maintenance of the system
6. Tax on the supply

The first four parts of that process were paid for many decades ago. We don't need to keep paying for them fifty years later. Item five includes the periodic replacement of equipment. This is where the costs are in the current system.

With item six, a considerable portion of what we pay for our energy is made up of taxes paid to the government. They did nothing for it but took the lion's share of the revenue. Does this seem fair to you, or does it sound like someone is taking the piss? When I say they do nothing to earn it, I forget to mention they created the monopoly (they call it legislation) to keep the whole mafia scam going.

If an outside party has centralized control over our energy supply, they can hold us to ransom. Heat and food are two of humans' foundational needs. It's easy to control a population if you control their basic needs, or in this case, their energy supply.

Did you know that over one billion people don't even have access to electricity? How could an electric vehicle future be possible if 20% of the population doesn't have electricity?

The end goal is to remove people from energy poverty. We can do this by making energy free or very low-cost. The two costs in this *'bridge'* solution are the initial infrastructure cost to build and distribute it and the ongoing maintenance or replacement cost.

I'm proposing that rather than taking what's offered from the current system, the only way out of this system is to create our own localized *'off-grid'* energy system. As with the rest of the topics in this book, I'm looking at this solution from the viewpoint of being an island in the middle of the ocean, so essentially, if rolled out, you'd have multiple *'islands'*, whether onshore or offshore, each being independent of one another, and independent of the centralized energy grid.

Every great solution needs a methodology or process to help us achieve that result. So, we look at this in three stages: *Reduce, Generate, and Manage.*

Reduce.

If we're on an island, we probably have a certain amount of energy demand to function daily. The idea with this first stage is to reduce that level of energy demand. We can do this by using alternative energy sources or different technologies. Suppose you decide to install a new heating system in your home. If your home only has single-glazed windows or no insulation in the walls, the *'energy demand'* will be much higher. You'd need to generate six times as much energy to achieve the same result. So, by reducing that demand first, you can reduce the size of the boiler that you need.

To reduce energy demand, you can upgrade the lighting to low energy, install new glazing, install a heat recovery ventilation system, & install insulation.

Suppose you're designing the building from scratch. In that case, you might design it to take advantage of crosswinds, for example, reducing the need for air conditioning in hot countries.

Likewise, in cold countries, say in northern Europe, you'd upgrade the thickness & quality of glazing in north-facing windows. Similarly, in warmer countries, you might reduce the impact of *'solar gain'*, which happens when the sun is shining on a window, causing the room to overheat, meaning you need to use air conditioning to reduce the temperature again to a comfortable level.

Other methods could be to look at alternative energy fuels. For example, an electric shower can be replaced with a boiler-fed shower instead. This is because an electric shower acts like a fast-acting kettle; it instantaneously heats a small amount of water, whereas the heated water is generated in bulk with a boiler-powered unit. When anything is generated at scale, it's cheaper to generate.

Following these principles, you can reduce energy demand in a standard building by 60-80%.

Generate

After you've reduced your energy needs, you can generate that *'need'* locally, either on-site or as part of a shared community energy source.

If we were using my island example, let's say we had some houses on the island, a hotel resort, some workspace buildings, & a small school. We could look at generating energy for each building individually. Still, it would be more efficient & cheaper to generate it at a central source and then distribute it to each building on the island. We've got to consider the cost of distributing it; if it's many miles of cabling or pipework, the price will be very high, and the *'energy loss'* in the system also increases with distance.

Besides being cheaper due to its scale, the beauty of a centralized distribution model is that everyone can share that resource. For example, with an individual building, you'd design the equipment to cover the *'energy demand'*, but some days, you might need a bit extra. To prevent running short, add additional capacity to that design. This means that if you don't use that capacity, it's wasted. With extra capacity comes extra cost because equipment has to be bigger, such as batteries, storage tanks, burner equipment, etc. But in a centralized model, another building can use any spare capacity & it doesn't go to waste. A centralized model offers much more flexibility in how that energy is used.

The type of technology you can use depends on where you're located in the world, & what natural resources you have available. If you're near the equator, solar energy is a good choice because you have an abundance of sun as a natural resource.

One caveat to that is solar panels have an optimum temperature range, so at the peak times of sun in a desert, for example, the solar panels may either reduce their operating efficiency or, over time, it can reduce the panel's life expectancy.

The most basic form of energy generation is what we've had for the last 100+ years. We can burn coal, wood, oil, or gas to generate energy. This isn't sustainable, as there's only a finite amount. We don't control its supply, and following this route, we never escape the energy slavery the system has created.

The other issue with distribution is that some energy is lost in that distribution network. The further away from its source, the more energy gets lost. There are many reasons behind this, from an increase in resistance levels in the case of electricity to heat loss from looking at a heat distribution pipework.

If considering a project, such as our island example, where buildings are spread across many miles, it may be more accessible and more beneficial to create multiple centralized generation units, which means you can still benefit from shared demand without the cost of distribution being unfeasibly high.

Biomass. If we cut down a tree & burn it to generate energy, we might get 2-3 weeks' worth of energy from that tree, yet it takes 40 years to grow it. In this case, is it a sustainable source of generation? Probably not. However, alternative biomass fuel sources, such as bamboo or hemp, grow faster than a tree. You do need a lot of space to grow this fuel source, and when grown, it'll need to be harvested & then processed before it can be burnt. These are all resource costs to be factored into the decision.

Wind. Depending on your level of demand and how windy it gets, the viability of using wind to provide electricity depends. The other issue with wind turbines is that they're ugly and only work well within defined wind speed parameters. If your site experiences extreme wind speeds, it can damage the turbine, so usually, it'll switch off if the wind reaches the turbine's limit.

Heat pumps. A heat pump takes heat from under the ground and brings it to the surface as heat/cooling for your building. There are two main types of systems: First, drilling a very deep vertical hole into the earth's core and then laying a pipe inside that hole. The second route is to lay a pipe inside a series of trenches in a horizontal formation across the ground.

With the first option, we must consider the viability of drilling a very deep hole underground. In our island example, it's probably not viable.

We need a vast ground area to lay the horizontal pipework for the second option. This area is forever out of bounds for future development, though you could probably build a golf course over it.

Air-source heat pumps work similarly, except they create heat/cooling from the air around them rather than the ground.

Solar PV. Solar PV can be used as glass-like sheets or, more recently, an alternative to traditional roof tiles. I've also heard whispers about the PV technology being integrated into standard window glazing. However, I've yet to see any real-life examples. I prefer to avoid seeing fields filled with these panels; they're ugly & they detract from the landscape. Suppose we use solar PV on a development project. In that case, we prefer to imagine a more innovative design, keeping them out of sight while performing a dual function.

Solar Thermal. Solar thermal panels are similar to Solar PV, but rather than generating electricity, they generate hot water. They contain several tubes, each heating up and feeding a hot water storage tank. From a visual perspective, they look very similar to a Solar PV panel.

Hydropower. Hydropower might be achievable if you're close to a running water source. Likewise, wave power can be used to generate electricity from the sea. Hydropower schemes have been created in many rural locations for dual purposes. The water source also provides the community with a water supply. Still, by collecting the water at its highest point through a dam, they generate electricity as it filters down to the community.

Hydrogen. I feel hydrogen will be a major catalyst for achieving energy Freedom. Whilst it's at its earliest stages of development now and is quite expensive, water is the most abundant natural resource on this planet, so finding a way to tap into that resource is good for us all. As technology develops, the price will reduce.

CHP (Combined Heat and power). It produces heat/cooling and power and is generated by burning a fuel source. Traditionally, the fuel source has been natural gas, but biomass is also starting to be used more frequently.

Anaerobic Digestion (waste to heat). What happens to all that waste you throw away every year? In many cases, it goes to landfill. Still, there's a solution where that waste, rather than going to landfills, is used to generate energy.

A community should consider whether we generate sufficient waste to provide the waste converter with enough fuel to power our energy demands. This option could indirectly incentivize us to create more waste so we don't run out of power.

It may work well for a business that produces waste as a by-product of its processes. Still, the image of people desperately seeking rubbish to keep the heating on doesn't sit well in the bigger *'Freedom for Humanity'* vision.

Free energy devices. As mentioned, many inventions have been suppressed, buried, and killed off over the last century. These inventions have started to come to light more recently, and people are working to create the free energy devices they were meant to be. I have a manual on how to make ten different free energy devices.

Biofuels. Biofuels are less of an energy generator technology but worth including as an alternative fuel source. We're now seeing many biofuel types emerging, including an equivalent fuel source for rockets and other aircraft, which typically need very high-octane fuels. Then, specialist fuels are created for motorsport and high-performance cars. However, one of the original biofuels is recycled vegetable oil from our local takeaways and chip fryers. This was big news twenty years ago but has gone quiet recently.

Batteries and fuel cells. If we're generating energy, there's a strong chance we won't have sufficient demand to use all of that energy when it's generated. In the past, this would have meant much of that energy being wasted, with Solar PV panels being the perfect example. Electricity is created during the day, but most of our electricity demand is at night when it's dark, and we need to use lighting and cooking equipment.

Creating an energy storage capability should be a big priority as part of the bigger energy strategy for any project. Various battery technologies are available, from old-school lead-acid batteries to lithium batteries. This is an area where a lot of development is happening, so anything I write about current technology now will probably be old news in six months.

Batteries and energy storage are where the most significant change will happen over the next few years.

We should also consider how we'll dispose of these items at the end of their life. Can we refurbish them so they don't need to be disposed of in the future?

Manage.
The third stage of the framework we call *'Manage'* includes how we use the system day-to-day, such as our behaviours. More importantly, it's about monitoring the equipment and its performance, maintaining it properly, and replacing items at the end of their lifespan.

Let's assume we've created an energy source for our island community. We've got some batteries to store that energy.

Those batteries might last ten years, so we need a plan to expand their useful lifespan through proper maintenance. Still, we want to avoid an unexpected cost ten years in the future to replace those batteries. Hence, as part of that plan, we pay into a *'replacement fund'* for that maintenance & replacement when it comes due. It's much easier to pay £100 per month now rather than £100,000 at an unknown date in the future. This fund model should be factored into any community business model.

The water options

The options for water are pretty simple, whilst also limited.

Reduce: The first thing to consider is whether we can reduce water demand. One way to do this is to cut back on our usage. One example is using water-less toilets.

I'm not saying these are the ideal solutions; I'm providing one example of reducing water demand. Every application will be different.

Reuse: The next option is recycling water. To do this, we use what's called *greywater recycling*. For example, we shower using fresh water. This shower water is filtered and stored before being used to flush the toilet. We can also use it to water our food garden. If done correctly, we can also use toilet water as fertilizer - called blackwater recycling. Still, to avoid outbreaks of typhoid, this should be done correctly.

Sources: Next, we need to look at our water sources. Rainwater collection from your roof space and other runoffs, such as along pathways, is the next natural source. If you can collect and store as much of this water as possible, this will reduce the amount of water we need from other sources.

The next *'rainwater catchment'* is creating swales
and dams in the landscape to catch and store water
naturally.

When all rainwater collection options are
exhausted, we need to look elsewhere. The first
option is to look at streams and rivers from which
we can take it. Before choosing this option,
investigate what's further upstream, as something
may contaminate your future water source. The
next is to drill a borehole. Drilling to a depth of 600
meters is essential, as water at shallower depths
contains toxins and runoff of chemicals from
neighbouring farms and industrial process plants.

One option in smaller communities and
island-based locations is to use a desalination plant,
where seawater is taken and the salt removed,
making it safe to drink. They take salt water from
the ocean and *'de-salt'* it through reverse osmosis,
removing the salt from the water to create drinking
water.

This all sounds great, considering the planet has so much salt water. Still, the problem is that the *'waste product'* from the desalination process is lots and lots of brine, which in most cases is pumped back into the ocean at massive concentrated levels. This high salt concentration kills all plant and animal life around it in that area, which causes underwater deserts. So, whilst the desalination process creates more than it consumes, it also has a harmful knock-on effect on the sealife, making it a non-sustainable process.

One final option I've seen used in arid desert environments is a system for trapping condensation. This system is too technical to describe in this book, but quite a few videos online explain it in more depth.

The final thing to consider is the parasites and bacteria in the water and how to remove them. There are numerous methods we can use to kill any unwanted bacteria.

On a small scale, we've got tablets that we can use to purify the water, making it safe to drink. Another method is adding chemicals, an option I don't like. We can also use special filters, such as UV filters, which *'zap'* any bacteria as they flow through the system. When I was an apprentice electrician in 1995, we worked with a construction company in rural parts of Scotland renovating ancient stone cottages.

Most of these cottages didn't have roads; we used a 4x4 off-road vehicle to reach them. The cottages were too far from civilization to be connected to the mains water supply, so most of the time, they had a private water supply, either from a borehole, a well or, more often, from a nearby stream. According to the *'experts'*, this water source would breed various parasites. Still, the interesting fact is that we never had to pump gallons of chlorine or fluoride into these streams. We fitted a basic ultraviolet filter in the cottage, which would *'zap'* any *'bad bacteria'* before it got into the house.

The waste options

One of the world's biggest problems is a need for more awareness about waste in our ecosystem. Some might say the blame lies with consumerism, but it's much easier than that. There are solutions available to us, but very few know about them because it's cheaper for the government to fill shipping containers with rubbish & send them to Asia. Much of this is common sense, but if you don't know it exists, well, you'll never understand there are better options available.

We first need to identify what comes into our ecosystem and what possible waste those items might produce. I note that some countries, Rwanda being one example, have placed a complete ban on bringing plastic bags into the country. It's illegal to bring a plastic bag into the country. Following a similar approach means when you've identified each item of potential waste, then understanding if you have a method of disposing of it.

Controlling whether anyone brings it into the ecosystem in the future will completely remove any future problems for your community.

In the UK, the brainless government believed the answer to the plastic bag problem was for supermarkets to charge people five pence for every plastic bag. This soon became another money-making scam, as the supermarkets dropped the cheaper five-pence bags and replaced them with bags costing sixty pence. It was the same bag but at a much higher price. It hasn't prevented the use of plastic bags. They failed to understand that people still use plastic bin liners, which are all still sent to landfill—acres and acres of black bin bags filled with rubbish.

Local councils in the UK have local 'recycling centres' where residents can take their old cardboard boxes and garden waste, etc. and put them into dedicated skips for recycling.

But one thing they haven't sorted is those electronic items that get thrown away. Until two years ago, much of this electronic waste was shipped to Ghana, which has the world's biggest landmass of electronics waste. Anything from TV screens to mobile phones to old Irons. The ground is so toxic the government has fenced most of it off to prevent the locals from scavenging through it. For decades, governments from all over the world have been illegally dumping this rubbish in Ghana.

The first step is auditing what comes into your ecosystem and identifying items based on their potential waste output. Next, we can consider the disposal methods for each type of waste.

Composting: Lots of what we dispose of can be composted. The general rule of composting is, *'If it's lived, it can be composted'*. So that means food waste, dead animals, animal faeces, plants, tree cuttings, cardboard, and even hair cuttings can be composted.

The composting process is generally very quick, with one method only taking a few weeks. One side benefit of composting is that the pile of decomposing waste gets very hot, so running a water pipe through the middle of the compost pile can mean that hot water is generated as the heat from the compost pile transfers into the water pipe. The composting process creates a nutrient-rich source of soil that can be reused within the community.

Pigs: Other waste disposal methods include feeding food waste to pigs. The pigs eat the waste and create lots of manure, which can then be placed on your food beds and increase the nutritional quality of your soil.

Reed beds: For toilet waste, we can use a reed bed system, whereby the waste is collected, and the reeds clean any toxins from it. This is also rich in nutritional sources for your soil.

Regular compost waste can also be added to your food beds, transferring all those nutritional sources back into the soil and helping the plants grow.

This combination of processes generally disposes about 95% of the waste within our ecosystem. By auditing what comes into the system & understanding which items can't be disposed of easily, we can either research specific ways to dispose of these items or prevent them from entering the ecosystem by using an alternative.

There are other ways of disposing of the waste, which I've not mentioned so far. Our governments use more archaic methods, like digging a hole and burying it. Otherwise, it could be burnt, but this isn't really a solution I like because of the toxic fumes it creates.

Earthship Construction: You can also construct buildings with waste materials.

For example, many examples exist of people building homes from old tyres packed with soil. Others are built from old glass bottles. If you inherit a site with lots of waste already there, an Earthship model could be the perfect opportunity to construct the community for free while solving the waste problem, too.

Paying for the infrastructure

We need to consider how we'll pay for all this new technology. Remember the end objective of free electricity? There are several more obvious options.

Community donation. This option involves the community donating a share of the initial development cost.

Community investment. Rather than donating money, certain community members each invest in the project.

The investment vehicle runs until the investment has been paid back to those funding members whilst also providing an annual dividend to each investor in the project until that payback is complete. Each energy user, or the community as a whole, pays for the energy they use.

The investment vehicle already exists today as an ESco (Energy Supply Company). The difference between this and the existing model is that when the initial project costs have been paid for, the cost of energy would reduce dramatically.

Revenue source. An alternative model is to create a revenue-generating source, such as building a hotel. This hotel generates a profit, which is used to pay for the initial development of the energy infrastructure and ongoing repair and maintenance, meaning that the community members don't pay anything for their energy usage.

Commercial loan. The downside of this option, over the others, is that every penny you spend to pay back the loan removes money from local circulation. The debt also carries interest. With the other options, the money stays circulating within the local community.

Locally invested returns. Using the investment returns of the community, as described in the formula chapter of the book, these investment returns are used to pay off the monthly cost, both infrastructure costs and ongoing management & repair costs.

In reality, the perfect solution will depend on the circumstances at the time, including whether your community has any money and whether they wish to invest it into such a project. The solution may be to use a combination of all these routes.

Mortal

In this chapter, we'll examine the elements related to the human body, including our health and the food sources we consume.

Health

The subject of health & how we improve it is an exciting topic. Around 98% of the population suffers from a severe lack of good health. We have already discussed the reasons behind that.

Now, we must look at some alternatives, first healing people's ailments and then considering how to prevent further ailments in the future.

I'm continually improving on this, but based on where my health was a decade ago, it's significantly better. Back then, my health was probably like that of the average person in the UK. Overweight, prescribed long-term pharmaceutical drugs, with a list of health issues that wouldn't go away. I'd had all kinds of scans & cameras inside me, but the Doctor didn't know what was wrong with me. Their only answer was that I'd have to keep increasing the dosage of each drug for the rest of my life.

By that point, I'd already stopped drinking alcohol after discovering I was gluten intolerant, but like everyone else my age, before that point, I'd go out every weekend; I'd drink two bottles of wine before I went out, followed by 25-30 spirits. I'm surprised my liver didn't give up on me.

Still, this path is very similar to most people in the UK, so it's considered normal behaviour.

The existing allopathic health system doesn't intend to fix the root cause; it only suppresses the symptom to make the patient believe the problem has gone away. Apart from emergency care, like dealing with a broken bone, we must rethink how we care for our bodies completely. This involves considering alternative forms of medicine and healing practices.

Routine detoxes are a couple of the practices I've adopted since I started improving my health. When I talk about detoxing to people, they have this strange idea that a detox is just removing meat from their diet for a day or two or that it's some method of losing weight. A real detox means purifying what goes in and removing any built-up waste already inside you.

This means doing water fasts. It needs to be pure water, not some toxic cocktail of chemicals your government provides to you. Why would you try detoxifying yourself by drinking chlorine & fluoride? It doesn't make any sense.

In addition, we also need to get rid of any built-up waste in the body, and I do this with an enema. Each month, I do a 24-hour water fast; every three months, a three-day water fast; and at least once every year, a seven-day water fast. Normally, I'll do an enema with every fast. During the fasting process, rather than using energy to digest food, the body uses that unspent energy to repair damaged cells & tissue.

Since I changed my health routine nine years ago, I haven't taken any pharmaceutical medications. During this time, I've suffered no recurrence of the original symptoms. I also feel a lot healthier and have a lot more energy.

Repair: We need to think about fixing our broken bodies. There's little point in visiting a spa for a massage if the reason for needing that massage isn't rectified first. The original intention of a spa was to use natural healing methods to cure the body's ailments. Over time, this has become more of an Instagram-worthy experience, where people sit around drinking prosecco & painting themselves in chocolate. It's become the opposite of the original intention for a spa experience. I'm not saying the experience makes the individual's health worse, but sitting around drinking alcohol doesn't help things.

This type of business has a great opportunity to return to the original intention of a spa. Many people will be searching for alternative healthcare methods, and these businesses can fill that need.

They can still feed the needs of the Instagram selfie crew but offer that as more of the *'luxury pampering'* offer rather than the foundational

282

treatment fixing the basic ailments of the people. This takes much more space than just having a treatment room & an indoor pool. International legacy brands, such as Six Senses, insist on having a minimum floor area of 1,000 square meters dedicated to the spa facility, which means a business has to be committed to providing a spa product for guests if they're to invest in this scale of infrastructure.

An upside to a business following this path is that it may attract a new clientele and generate additional revenue streams. Suppose the company is a day spa without hotel facilities. In that case, there's a clear opportunity to add the foundational treatments to the spa offering along with bedrooms, a restaurant, and other income generating product lines.

Coming onto actual treatments for the restoration process, we can dig much deeper into all kinds of alternative therapies, from Reiki to Ayurvedic practices.

We can also include plant medicine ceremonies with Ayahuasca & Iboga. Many of these alternative natural remedies have been around for centuries. For example, in South America, Tobacco is a sacred healing medicine. It's strange how everything we've been told about things like tobacco and cannabis by Western society, these are all-natural products. Still, we're brainwashed into believing they're bad for us. It's not the tobacco that's bad for us; it's the tar they add to it that kills us.

Our indigenous ancestors knew how to heal themselves. Nature has answers for everything, staring us in the face. Take nettles as an example; beside every patch of nettles is also a patch of dock leaves. Many plants and herbs that we grow in our garden can heal us. Other natural healing methods might be tissue salts or aromatherapy oils. Everything has its application.

One of the leading causes of our ailments is what goes into our bodies, both food and environmental stress.

We can also affect our health based on our thoughts and psychological conditioning. Did you know that some people are fat because subconsciously, they're crying out to *be seen* by the world? Hence, their bodies take on the task of making themselves as big as possible to make them *'seen'*.

Another example is what we tell ourselves. Have you ever noticed that when someone is diagnosed with a terminal disease & provided a life expectancy timeframe, the majority of people die almost in the exact time they've been told? Still, occasionally, an individual will reject the diagnosis & far exceed the time expectations given.

I know two individuals this happened to. The first was given three months to live but was still alive seven years later. The second was given six months but died five years later.

The reason why has been proven across many experiments, where it was discovered that what we tell ourselves becomes true. Our thoughts and our words create our reality.

Another major cause of health issues is food intolerance. There are seven foods which most people have an intolerance to. When I say intolerance, I mean their body cannot digest them, so it creates all kinds of illnesses, diseases, and sickness symptoms. Gluten, Dairy, Eggs, Soya, Nuts, Sugar & Salt. 70% of the population has some form of intolerance or allergy to at least one of these. Whilst they might not realize it, the symptoms can be anything from feeling lethargic, having acid reflux, headaches, migraines, false diagnosis of IBS (irritable bowel syndrome), or even joint pains. The problem is your body cannot digest these substances if you're intolerant to them, so your body stores them as fat, & over time, they start to grow tumours.

When I learnt about my intolerances, I lost twenty kilograms in two months just by not eating foods that contained these ingredients. The medical system will not show these as an intolerance. When the Doctor tested me for gluten, the test result came back negative. This is because they test for an allergy rather than an intolerance. A gluten allergy is called celiac disease; if you eat gluten as a celiac, you'll probably die. Eating gluten when you're intolerant will cause migraines, breathing issues & numerous other unconnected symptoms. There's a big difference.

Do you think it's any coincidence that natural health practitioners, & other *'non-allopathic'* alternatives have been outlawed? In some jurisdictions, they carry a prison sentence & even the death penalty. These *'natural healers'* have been presented to the world as *'crazy'* or practising satanic witchcraft just for mixing a few natural herbs in a bowl. It's only in the past few years that things like Cannabis have been made legal under strict conditions.

Those strict conditions create a way for the system to tax its sale & usage. The only reason most drugs are made illegal is because the government cannot tax them when someone grows the plant in their own home. The other reason is that the traditional medical industry would collapse if everyone had access to all the alternative medicines and natural healing techniques.

Blue zone principles

If you've not heard of the blue zones before, these are locations around the world where large portions of the population live to over 100 years old. It's said this is because the inhabitants of each blue zone area live their lives by following certain principles, which I'll share below. These principles are a lifestyle choice conducive to a long, healthy life. These principles must be adopted within every community development.

The blue zone principles are:

Move naturally: They don't run marathons or spend their life in a gym. They live in areas that require movement without thinking about it, such as growing a food garden, so they get regular exercise every time they enter their garden.

Purpose / ikigai: Each person has a sense of purpose, a reason why they wake up in the morning

Downshift: They follow routines to get rid of stress

80% rule: Eat the smallest meal in late afternoon and early evening. Only eating until they're 80% full, and never eating to a point where they feel full.

Plant slant: Eating a mainly plant-based diet, eating meat on average only five times per month

Wine @ 5: Drinking alcohol moderately but regular. Drinking 1-2 glasses every day

Belong: Belonging to & following a faith or sense of togetherness.

Loved ones first: keeping family close, including parents and grandparents, having a life partner, and investing time with their children.

Right tribe: Being around the right social circle, a group that promotes healthy behaviours

These nine principles can improve our life expectancy by 10-12 years. By designing our environment along these principles, community residents don't have to *'try'* to live the blue zone way; they live it naturally as it's the only way for them to be.

We can do this very simply, for example, by having sports facilities such as tennis courts, swimming pools & golf courses.

We can have a communal food garden & build public paths in areas that naturally increase the heart rate. Areas for meditation, yoga & martial arts can be an easy way to de-stress, & developing our community with multi-generational living in mind means that all generations are close to one another, again promoting the principle of being close to loved ones.

Food

If you're under the illusion that anything you eat from mainstream food sources is good for you, I've got some devastating news. Everything you eat from the supermarket or the fast food takeaway harms your health.

Take the well-known fast food chain. Its burgers aren't even made of real meat. They're lab-grown to taste like meat. It's time to start questioning what we're putting in our bodies.

With all the chemicals sprayed over our foods, it's no wonder people are sick and full of disease. To be healthy, we need to start with what we put in our mouths: food and drink. Different climates and soil types determine what we can grow and when. We'll also need alternative growing areas, such as sheltered polytunnels or greenhouses. Some people also use heated areas for growing food through the cold season.

We also want to maximize the efficiency of our food production. We've already looked at sacred geometry as a method to increase production yields. Another method is electroculture.

Electroculture works by picking up electricity in the atmosphere around us and grounding it by making it flow through our food beds. People typically see yields of 2-3x their average growth rate by adopting the electroculture principles.

Regarding space requirements, if we use raised beds for growing, again dependent on soil fertility, we need around 300 square feet per person to produce enough vegetables for one person to survive throughout the year. Adding fruit and any meat sources will increase the size requirement.

We'll need incubator space like a potting shed or greenhouse for growing seeds, and we'll also want to create storage facilities and a preparation area. Hence, a root cellar is a good option for storage, as it prevents sunlight and heat from reaching the food. Many people use canning to store food for the winter period. Still, storing it in glass jars is better, as it prevents the metals from the can from leaching into the food.

So, our community plan includes a food garden, an alternative health spa, and all of the blue zone principles.

Know thyself

One of my passions is having a vision, & seeing that vision come to life. This is probably why I've always had a love for property development. If I have everything I need in my life, I'm not bothered about money; my ultimate intention is to create something beautiful, whether it's a lovely house, a hotel resort, or a village that ties everything in this book together under a single project. Seeing that vision come to life is what I like, but it goes much deeper than this. The creation process is just a tool I've been given to achieve a much deeper purpose.

It's like this book. Any income I receive from selling this book will be tiny compared to the 1200+ hours I've invested into writing it and the lifetime of learning it. I'm not writing it with the intention of *'chasing money'*; I'm doing it because I have a vision for a better way of living outside of the authoritarian government systems, & I want to share that vision by providing a roadmap to get there.

I share these ideas and thoughts to put the call out—the call to those who resonate with the message so we can do it together. The book intends to bring like-minded souls together.

But the problem with most people is that they aren't on their true path. When we aren't on our destined path, we do two things. First, we climb other people's ladders, believing it's our own. What I mean by this is that we're easily influenced by society, our families, and so-called gurus, thinking we should copy their exact *formula for success*. We make career choices based on what others believe is best for us.

In other cases, we get sucked into the latest get-rich-quick scheme. How many people have been sucked into property investing, forex trading, buying businesses, crypto, NFTs, or Multi-level marketing scams in the last 15 years?

This might be their path for a small portion, but for the rest, they're chasing the lifestyle of that person selling the dream. The few who fight their way up the ladder discover it's not what they want and doesn't make them happy. But most people spend decades trying to climb that ladder, never moving any closer to the desired finish line.

The second route some take when they aren't on their true path is to turn to the *dark side'*, Whether that be a blatant crime or just having the intent to screw people over. I've been screwed over a lot by people I've worked with; these were people I trusted. But if people were on the right path, they wouldn't need to choose these options.

A few weeks ago, I received an email from someone trying to blackmail me for money. I suspect it was the same scam this individual plays on everyone. Anyone else might have just complied with the demands *'to make the problem go away'*, but in my case, I knew his blackmail wasn't true.

He'd requested I send him £1,500 in Bitcoin within 48 hours, or else he'd share a video of me, apparently masturbating to porn. I thought, wow, imagine what a treat the ladies would have if they watched that. But after my initial excitement, I realized it wasn't true - I hadn't watched porn for over fifteen years. You can imagine my disappointment after realizing this.

In the USA, there are two million people in the prison system. Similar statistics are shared across most countries worldwide. If everyone were on their path, there would be almost no crime—at least, no crime originating from the desire to get money and possessions.

The majority of people don't like their jobs. If you go to work with the sole intention of getting money, that's called slavery. Work, generally speaking, isn't slavery.

But, when you exchange your time for money, doing something you don't want to do, that's slavery. Still, worst of all, you're enslaving yourself.

If you ever get that *'Monday morning feeling'*, it's your soul telling you to change something. Figuring out what that *'thing'* is—maybe it's the people, maybe it's the boss, perhaps you're just not fulfilled, or you're bored—is probably your starting point to realizing this is not your path.

In my career, I think I've always been on my path; it's just that sometimes, I probably stayed too long on one section of that path, which caused me a lot of internal stress. This always boiled down to deep unhappiness, even though I didn't understand why.

Why are you here? I wouldn't have known why I was here if you'd asked me twenty years ago.

Still, I knew it had to be something more meaningful than just bidding for, & delivering contracts in our business at the time. Just the thought that I'd repeat the same basic process the rest of my life, day after day, week after week, year after year. Was this really what I was put on this planet to do? That's where my inner discomfort was rooted, the thought that I'd repeat that same pattern every year for 50 years, and then I'd die. There has to be more to life than the hamster wheel existence.

My biggest problem at the time was that nobody around me saw this as a problem themselves. They were happy to do this for the rest of their life - they couldn't understand why I wouldn't want this for myself, too.

The path we walk gives us the tools needed to fulfil our purpose. Those skills I've learned during my life and those jobs I've done are the tools; they're not the purpose. It is like going through an apprenticeship. We learn the skills that we'll use later on. We go through these different experiences to mould ourselves into the person we need to be to fulfil our mission.

When someone performs a particular role in life believing this is their purpose, I don't believe that role is the actual purpose. Let me give you an example. Imagine someone who is an excellent public speaker; they've practised and perfected their talks and travel worldwide, and their words touch people's souls. They might believe this to be their purpose. I'd go further than that. Their public speaking ability is just their tool; it's their vehicle. Their actual purpose is to spread a message. For a motivational speaker, that message might push people into their true path. The medium is not the message; it's just the channel for that message.

I am still trying to discover a clear path to finding your purpose. The universe has probably dropped clues in your path for a while, and you've either ignored them or flat-out dismissed them. I can share the junction points I've encountered to help me identify mine.

One system I'd recommend to help with this is a profiling system called *Human Design*. This system is unique to everyone. I'm a *'6/2 mental projector'* with a *'left angle cross of defiance'*.

Unless you've studied the system, this will mean nothing. Still, in simple terms, it provides an insight into my purpose and how I fulfil it.

Interestingly, it all relates to everything I've done and what I've been passionate about for over two decades.

I'm here to help create a new future for humanity, free from the current systems, by being a role model and guide to others, all based on sharing my experiences. Writing this book is one step toward doing that.

The next area to consider, which may help you get on the right path, is what you're inspired to do. What would you most like to do if you didn't have to go to work every day? What type of TV programmes do you most like watching & why? What are your interests? If you could do one thing for the rest of your life without being paid for it, what would that be? Every time you do something, ask yourself this question.

I've always had a passion for property development. I love seeing something transform, and my visions come to life. I've been around this industry my whole life; I was born into it, as my parents, grandparents, and great-grandparents have all been in it their entire lives.

My other passion, which has always been smouldering in the background and driving me behind the scenes, is a quest for Freedom & travel. At its basic level, I always rebel against people telling me what to do - whether that be an authority figure, a client, or the government; & I've lived or worked in most towns & cities around the UK, but I always have the drive to create businesses in other countries. I love experiencing new cultures & I probably have more international friends than those from the UK.

In 2015, I volunteered with a charity that supported people experiencing homelessness in the West Midlands, UK. In this charity, we'd take out food and drink to people living on the streets of Wolverhampton. As part of that project, I decided to dedicate a week of my time to help one of the homeless people get back into work, back into society, and off the streets. We'd set up a house for him, and I walked the streets of Wolverhampton, talking to every business, trying to find him a job.

The problem was, whilst he was grateful for me setting this up for him, he didn't want it. He didn't want to be part of traditional society.

I couldn't understand it then, but he was happy just as he was. I've realized it's because he's achieved Freedom from the system. Living on the streets and begging for spare change might not be my idea of Freedom, but it is one form of Freedom, and he was happy with it.

I've used an online tool called *'The Passion Test'*. I recommend trying it yourself. This tool helps you identify your top five general passions. Not surprisingly, if you look at my profile on the platform, you'll see that my number one passion is Freedom. You can find the assessment on the geniusu.com platform.

There's a role for everyone in society. That role might be taking care of the kids. It might be managing projects. Some people are naturally gifted at specific roles. They find these roles more enjoyable, & easier to do than others. If we created a utopian society, we'd need all types of natural skill sets. Where would we live if we didn't have a naturally skilled builder? The builder can only build a house if someone looks after his kids. And how would everyone eat if we didn't have someone to grow or cook food?

While a job might feel like slavery to one person, to another, it is a meditative process. Our problem as a society is that many people are stuck performing roles they hate to *'get money'* at the end of the week.

If everyone followed the paths they were passionate about, this dynamic would shift, and everyone would be happy working in roles they enjoyed.

Suppose you can make an inventory of all your skills, those things you do, and the experiences you enjoy. In that case, these are the tools you'll use to fulfil your purpose, just like our example of the motivational speaker. These skills aren't necessarily things you do a lot of. Add this to your skills inventory list.

If I rewind twenty years, I always enjoyed creating new service offerings for our business. We created less than three new service offerings every year, but I was responsible for creating these. In total, I spent between 50-100 hours creating each new service offering, which was time spent when I didn't have anything else to do. I remember thinking this was something I'd enjoy doing full-time.

Still, it comprised a tiny portion of my time with the rest of the business, managing projects and keeping clients satisfied.

Suppose you've ever taken a personality profiling test. In that case, you'll probably agree that 99% of them don't give you a life pathway. They tend to put you in a box and leave you feeling slightly disappointed—a sense of *that's great, but what now? How can I use this information to move forward?'*

Wealth Dynamics, created by Roger Hamilton, is one system that provides a useful pathway. The system works on the premise that there are eight core types of people. Each type has an entirely different pathway to success in their life in a way that's natural for them. For some, it's about shining a spotlight on others; people like Oprah Winfrey have done so successfully her whole career. For others, it's about seeing the future and creating a product or business to align with it.

People like Elon Musk, Walt Disney, & Richard Branson share this personality type. This is my personality type, too.

Whilst most people hear the title *'wealth dynamics'* & get put off by it, thinking it relates to managing your money, as Roger says, *'wealth is what you're left with after all the money is taken away'*. As Einstein once said, *'Everybody is a genius. But if you judge a fish by its ability to climb a tree, it will live its whole life believing it's stupid*. Wealth Dynamics is about first learning that you're a fish, then building on those natural strengths instead of living your entire life following someone else's success strategy.

Although we don't realize it, we all have a combination of twelve fundamental unconscious beliefs that drive our actions every day. These beliefs were imprinted on us in our first seven years of childhood. They run most people's lives if you're unaware of them. Unfortunately, we can't get rid of them, but if we're aware of them, we can learn to notice when we might be about to sabotage something in our lives.

Have you ever noticed how some people repeat specific patterns repeatedly?

Until a few years ago, I'd spent my whole career repeating the same unconscious pattern. The situation was different every time, but the outcome was always the same. Something just clicked when I learnt about these twelve fundamental beliefs driving us, and it made perfect sense. My whole life has been dedicated to seeking validation & approval from my Dad. When I learnt that, I instantly thought about the times I'd tell my Dad about a business idea, only to ask for his approval. Every business, project, idea, and life experience has been a way for me to receive his recognition, approval, or validation.

The problem is, if these subconscious beliefs are driving us, we'll never get what we're looking for because if that ever happened, it would shatter our subconscious belief, so our mind makes us do something to sabotage it before we reach that magical point.

So imagine spending your whole life trying to gain validation from someone else & constantly failing. The sad thing is, while trying to fill this hole, you never get to where your soul truly wants to go.

Whilst you can't get rid of these beliefs, you can be aware of them. Every time you make a decision, or if you have a vision for something in your life, if you're aware of these beliefs driving your thoughts, you can begin to notice whether you do want that *'thing'* or whether it's your subconscious beliefs trying to fill a hole. If you're interested in learning more about this, please enrol in a course called *'Create your destiny'* by William Whitecloud.

Education

Today's kids leave school with a lot of *'fake knowledge'*, memorized from textbooks, inverted fractions, and the like. Still, they lack the basic life skills that every human needs to function in this world.

This book isn't a go-to resource suggesting a step-by-step path to changing the education system, but we must throw out the current system and start again. I'm not blaming the teachers. I know many teachers who complain about the education system and how stupid it is. Still, they're forced to deliver the curriculum that's put in front of them. Many of the teachers I know have already left the teaching profession because they were so frustrated by it not delivering for a large proportion of the students.

We must start by giving each student or person a tailored learning program. Each person receives the foundational skills of reading, writing, basic math, basic English, and maybe some science, but also life skills, such as how to grow your food source, how to cook, how to solve problems, & how to communicate. After we've grasped the basics, we can focus on a lifelong learning approach.

Instead of sitting in a classroom for years, we spend one day every week dedicated to learning a subject we're interested in, all based on a particular goal we want to attain.

In addition to having one day a week dedicated to learning, we could also have a mentor in the subject matter: someone who has already walked the path we want to follow. These people may be like the elders of the community. If we don't learn from the generations before us, the human race will never evolve to the next level. We'll continue to start from zero and make the same repeated mistakes over and over again.

Wouldn't this be a better learning system, especially when we transition from 100% classroom-based learning to a method of learning by immersing ourselves in the chosen subject? That's how humans are designed to learn. We're not robots, so why would we learn like a robot?

Conclusion - Using the framework in your own life

Throughout these pages, we've highlighted some of the most nefarious acts of evil committed against the human race for more than a century. It doesn't matter whether you follow my suggestions; the objective is to free yourself from the current systems by becoming less reliant on them.

I've given you a framework to do that. Whilst I took the approach of a business model, creating a whole new functioning society outside of the traditional systems, everything comes down to replacing their systems with one of your own. If you want a pint of milk, you can buy it from the supermarket or get your own dairy cow. This is the extreme option, but it's just one easy example of shifting outside the system and becoming less reliant on it. You're much harder to control when you're less reliant on it.

I've shared some ideas for potential solutions around these issues. Still, some might find them overwhelming and wonder where best to start. I suggest one action you can take to begin that transformation process. Any change can seem daunting for most people, especially if it's a new path and you only have limited evidence of people doing it successfully.

Everything starts with you. Nobody is coming to save you. Nobody is going to change things for you. Donald Trump being reelected as president is not going to change anything. The *'white hats'* are not coming to save you, despite all that false hope spread among the new age community. Nothing changes unless you change it. Stop relying on someone else to come & fix it for you. Get off your arse and do something yourself for the sake of your family.

I'd suggest working with others, teaming up, collaborating, and partnering. This will make the task less daunting, and you'll all make progress together.

The model I've shared can be used on a micro level, but it can also be used on a macro level. It starts with one part of your own life, then your business, if you have one; your employer's business, if not; and your community, your county, your region, state, or country.

It very quickly becomes a movement that takes over the whole world. But it all starts with step one, your own life. Everything from that point on is just a domino effect.

If everyone focused on alternative options for their lives, the rest of the world would self-organize to accommodate that new way of being. No effort would be required. A business, a community, or a country is just a group working to achieve a shared objective, a shared culture.

Focus on working through one area of the book at a time. Dedicate time and resources to making that area its optimum state, starting with a review of where you are now, creating a vision of where you want to go, creating a plan to make it come to life, and then taking the necessary actions.

If you want to access unique content or hear about the latest opportunities, projects or businesses I'm involved with, I'd encourage you to join my VIP club. It's free, and you can join it by signing up at my website, www.wayne-fox.co.uk

About the author

Wayne Fox is a business re-ignitor, industry disruptor, commercial property developer, futurist, best-selling Author, & investor. Director of the Enyaw group, a UK-based investment firm that invests in *'freedom lifestyle'* ventures. He is experienced in achieving 7 & 8-figure revenue growth across previous SME ventures.

My online links:

Wayne Fox Website: www.wayne-fox.co.uk

Enyaw Group: www.enyawgroup.com

Enyaw Capital: www.enyawcapital.com

Enyaw Property: www.enyawproperty.co.uk

Linkedin:https://www.linkedin.com/in/waynefoxuk

Twitter: https://twitter.com/WayneFoxUK1

Instagram:https://www.instagram.com/waynefoxuk

Youtube:https://www.youtube.com/@WayneFoxUK

Udemy:https://www.udemy.com/user/wayne-fox-6